THE SHAMBHALA GUIDE TO YOGA

THE SHAMBHALA GUIDE TO YOGA

Georg Feuerstein

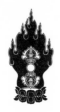

SHAMBHALA

Boston & London

1996

Shambhala Publications, Inc.
Horticultural Hall
300 Massachusetts Avenue
Boston, Massachusetts 02115
www.shambhala.com

Drawings in chapter 5 by Vicky MacDonald

9   8   7   6   5   4

Printed in the United States of America.
⊛ This edition is printed on acid-free paper that meets the
American National Standards Institute Z39.48 Standard.
Distributed in the United States by Random House, Inc., and
in Canada by Random House of Canada Ltd

Library of Congress Cataloging-in-Publication Data

Feuerstein, Georg.
    The Shambhala guide to yoga / Georg Feuerstein. — 1st ed.
      p.   cm.
    ISBN 1-57062-142-X(alk. paper)
    1. Yoga.   I. Title.
    BL1238.52.F48   1996   95-23896
    181'.45—dc20   CIP

Contents

Preface

The sage yoked in Yoga soon attains the Absolute (brahman).
—BHAGAVAD-GITA V.6

I have been studying the Yoga tradition since the early 1960s, and I continue to be awed by its enormous wealth of experience and understanding of the human condition. My own life has been deeply, lastingly, and benignly affected by the combined wisdom of the great teachers of Yoga, past and present. I have also seen the beneficial influence of Yoga practice in the lives of many others. I believe that this ancient and vast tradition is as relevant today as it was thousands of years ago, possibly more so.

All my various books on Yoga and other aspects of Indian spirituality have served one purpose: to make the genuine traditions available and accessible to those who are dissatisfied with watered-down Western derivatives and who wish to become informed about the authentic original teachings. The present book, too, is in alignment with this overall purpose of my life's work, which was first conceived and articulated in my late teens.

Each of my books is an attempt to offer yet another perspective on India's spiritual traditions. In the present book, I am providing an overview of the essentials of Yoga—understood not as a system of calisthenics but as a full-fledged spiritual tradition—that can both broaden and deepen the understanding of beginning students as well as serve as a compass for more advanced practitioners. I have singled out Classical Yoga and Tantra-Yoga (including Hatha-Yoga) for more detailed discussion, because these two branches of the Yoga tradition are of the greatest interest to Western students but are still often badly misunderstood.

I am very grateful to Samuel Bercholz and the editorial team of Shambhala Publications for inviting me to write this guide to Yoga. Working on this book gave me the opportunity to delve again into my favorite Sanskrit scriptures and to listen to the clarifying and inspiring thoughts of masters like Yajnavalkya, Patanjali, Vyasa, Gaudapada, Shankara, Ashtavakra, Gheranda, Svatmarama Yogindra, Swami Vivekananda, Sri Aurobindo, Swami Sivananda, Ramana Maharshi, Swami Nikhilananda, Swami Muktananda, and Nisargadatta Maharaj. I have quoted them whenever possible.

May this book bring understanding (*vijnana*), wisdom (*jnana*), and joy (*sukha*)! *Aum tat sat.*

—Georg Feuerstein

Georg Feuerstein established the Yoga Research Center to conduct and promote literary and comparative research on Yoga; serve as a clearinghouse for medical, psychological, and other scientific data on Yoga; educate the public about all branches and aspects of Yoga through *Yoga World* newsletter, other publications, and seminars. For more information write to: Georg Feuerstein, Yoga Research Center, P. O. Box 1386, Lower Lake, CA 95457.

A Note on Pronunciation

Sanskrit words and names in this book are rendered according to a simplified system of transliteration commonly used in nonscholarly literature. The reader's attention is drawn to two spellings in particular:

The spelling *c* indicates the sound *ch*, as in *church*, in words such as *cakra*, *citta*, and the like.

The spelling *ch* indicates an aspirated *ch* sound, similar to the *ch-h* in *beach-house*; hence, *Chandogya-Upanishad*.

The spelling *sh* is used for both the retroflex ṣ and the palatal ś, with the following exceptions. The letter *s* alone is used in the title *Sri* (pronounced *shree*) for names such as *Sri Aurobindo* and *Sri Ramakrishna*, and in the name *Sivananda* (pronounced *Sheeva-nunda*).

THE SHAMBHALA GUIDE TO YOGA

1
Introducing Yoga

Evenness (samatva) *is called Yoga.*
—BHAGAVAD-GITA II.48

Yoga as Unitive Discipline

From the broadest possible perspective, all the various yogic approaches—and there are many—have the same overall purpose. That purpose is to help the spiritual practitioner transcend the ego-personality, or "lower" self, so that he or she may realize the "higher" Reality, whether it is conceived as the transcendental Self or as the Divine (God or Goddess). This spiritual realization is not necessarily understood in the same way by the various branches of Yoga. However, even though the schools of Yoga may differ in their preferred method and also in their interpretation of the nature of ultimate spiritual realization, all these differences can be regarded as creative variations on the same fundamental theme: They all are designed to lift the individual out of his or her ordinary perception of, and relationship to, the world.

How we perceive things determines how we relate to them, and, in turn, how we relate to things feeds back into our perception of them. In other words, there is a close relationship between our

1

thoughts and actions, or our attitudes and behavior. Thus, if we perceive a situation to be threatening, we are apt to fight or take flight. The Sanskrit texts employ the classic example of a person running away from a snake when in reality it is only a rope. On the other hand, if a child thinks of a stranger as kind or well-meaning, he or she is likely to respond to the stranger with a trust that may prove misplaced or even fatal. Similarly, if we look upon the world as a vale of tears, as did the Romantics, we are apt to behave in ways quite different from staunch philosophers of social progress and utopian optimism.

Finally, if we truly understand that our material life is inherently limited and that the pleasures we can derive from our body and mind are likewise limited, merely temporary, and certainly not ultimately fulfilling, then we can open ourselves to the possibility of a new perception: that happiness is independent of our nervous system and the stimuli that can excite it. This is indeed the great message of all forms of Yoga: Happiness is our essential nature, and our perpetual quest for happiness is fulfilled only when we realize who we truly are. This realization is an awakening to our Selfhood, which transcends the body-mind, the ego-personality, and the horizon of the world reflected in our ordinary experience. All this, and more, is captured in the word *yoga*.

The term *yoga* is a common word in the Sanskrit language—the language in which most of the Yoga scriptures are written. It also happens to be one of the most versatile Sanskrit terms, having a whole range of meanings that extend from simple "union" to "team," "constellation," and "conjunction." It is derived from the verbal root *yuj*, meaning "to harness, yoke, prepare, equip, fasten."

The male practitioner of Yoga is known as a *yogin* (or *yogi* in the nominative case) and the female practitioner as a *yogini*. Frequent synonyms are *yoga-vid* ("knower of Yoga") and *yukta* ("yoked one"). Sometimes the word *yoga-yuj* ("one who is yoked in Yoga") is used.

A master of Yoga may be referred to as a *yoga-raj* ("king of Yoga") or *yogendra* (from *yoga* and *indra*, meaning "lord").

In addition to *yoga* and *yukta*, the verbal root *yuj* also yields the old Sanskrit word *yuga*, denoting "yoke," which is the literal yoke placed upon an ox and the yoke or burden of the years. It is probably in the latter, metaphoric sense that *yuga* is applied to the four great world cycles, which according to Hinduism, continuously revolve, thus creating history. At present we are thought to be in the final world age, the *kali-yuga*, in which spirituality and morality are at their lowest ebb. The *kali-yuga* is the Dark Age, which is destined to terminate in a convulsive cataclysm, accompanied by a major purging of humanity. Thereafter a new Golden Age will begin, starting the four-phase cycle all over again.

The term *yoga* is closely related to a number of words in various Indo-European languages, including the English *yoke*, the German *Joch*, and the Latin *iugum*, which all have the same meaning. In a spiritual context, the word *yoga* can have two principal meanings. It can stand for either "union" or "discipline." In most instances, both connotations are present when the term *yoga* is used. Thus *dhyana-yoga* is the unitive discipline of meditation; *samnyasa-yoga* is the unitive discipline of renunciation; *karma-yoga* is the unitive discipline of self-transcending action; *kriya-yoga* is the unitive discipline of ritual; *bhakti-yoga* is the unitive discipline of love and devotion to the Divine, and so on.

What does *unitive* mean here? It describes Yoga's disciplined approach to simplifying one's consciousness and energy to the point where we no longer experience any inner conflict and are able to live in harmony with the world. More specifically, *unitive* refers to the goal of many branches and schools of Yoga, which is to realize our essential nature, the Self (*atman*, *purusha*), by consciously uniting with it. This understanding of Yoga is characteristic of those teachings that subscribe to a nondualist metaphysics according to which the Self is the ultimate singular Reality underlying all phenomena.

A different understanding prevails in the dualist schools, notably Patanjali's *yoga-darshana* ("vision/system of Yoga"), which is also known as Raja-Yoga or Classical Yoga. For Patanjali, the yogic process is not so much one of union with an ultimate Reality as disunion (*viyoga*), or disconnection, from the ego-personality. But the final outcome is the same, for when the spiritual practitioner has succeeded in transcending the ego, he or she simultaneously realizes the Self, or Spirit.

Is Yoga then a form of religion or mysticism? It is not possible to give a simple answer to this question, because the Yoga tradition is vast and complex and includes many approaches, some of which even contradict each other when viewed from an outward perspective. Thus it comprises schools that espouse total renunciation (*samnyasa*) and those that insist on the proper performance of one's obligatory works (*karman*) in the world; schools that regard dispassionate wisdom (*jnana*) as the only means to spiritual freedom and Self-realization and those that place love and devotion (*bhakti*) above all other methods; and schools that favor a complicated ritualism and those that preach the path of methodless spontaneity (*sahaja*).

Some branches and schools of Yoga are more religious, entailing elaborate ceremonies, temple worship, and sect membership; others are more mystical, focusing on individual renunciation and meditation. Perhaps the most appropriate label for all of them is *spirituality*: Yoga is India's particular brand of spirituality, and its constituent branches and schools share a common origin and a broad history that covers the remarkable span of five thousand years.

Just as the branches of a tree are attached to a single stem, the diverse strands within Yoga are all connected to a basic stock of ideas and practices. In fact, there is considerable theoretical and practical overlap between schools, and in many cases only a slight shift of emphasis demarcates one school from another. Also, even within one school a variety of opinions may be present, as teachers develop their own explanations on the basis of their scriptural interpretations and personal experiences. What unites these schools and branches of Yoga is their overarching goal, which is Self-realization.

The teachers of Yoga speak of this Self-realization as liberation (*moksha, mukti, apavarga, kaivalya*), awakening (*bodha, bodhana, bodhi, jagrat*), wisdom (*jnana, vidya, prajna*), independence/freedom (*svatantrya*), perfection (*siddhi*), or extinction (*nirvana*). And they provide many names for the ultimate Reality that is realized by the adept, including Supreme (*para*), Supreme Self (*parama-atman*), Supreme Object (*parama-artha*), Absolute (*brahman*), Being (*sat*), Nonbeing (*Asat*), Awareness/Consciousness (*cit, citi, cetana, samvid*), Bliss (*ananda*), God (*deva*), Goddess (*devi*), Lord (*ish, isha, ishvara*), Infinity (*ananta*), Full/Fullness (*purna, purnata*), Void/Voidness (*shunya, shunyata*), Light (*jyotis, prakasha*), Immortality (*amritatva, amarata*), and Unborn (*aja*).

A Bird's-Eye View of the History of Yoga

No one knows exactly when the Yoga tradition began. What is certain is that it was already considered ancient at the time of the *Bhagavad-Gita* (Lord's Song), the most popular of all Yoga scriptures, composed some twenty-five hundred years ago. Evidence of yogic beliefs and practices can be seen in the archaic *Rig-Veda* (Knowledge of Praise), which is the fountainhead of the sacred heritage of Hinduism. The *Rig-Veda*, consisting of 1,028 hymns composed in archaic Sanskrit, has recently been dated back to the third millennium BCE and earlier, which makes it the oldest literary document in any Indo-European language.

The Vedic hymns—the word *veda* means "knowledge"—are the inspired creations of seer-poets (*kavi*), whose spiritual discipline enabled them to look beyond the ken of the five senses and the sense-bound mind. These hymns are the distillate of their visionary experiences, ecstasies, and mystical insights and are traditionally regarded as revealed wisdom. All subsequent sages and religious thinkers within the fold of Hinduism, to one degree or another, based themselves on the Vedic revelation (*shruti*). Those who did not, like Gautama the Buddha and Vardhamana Mahavira, the founder of Jainism, were considered to stand outside the pale of Hinduism. The *Rig-Veda* is one of four Vedic hymnodies, the other three being the *Yajur-Veda*, the *Sama-Veda*, and the *Atharva-Veda*. They are rich depositories of early Indian spirituality, which we may style a form of archaic Yoga.

A variety of yogic motifs are also depicted on the artifacts of the Indus-Sarasvati civilization, which flourished in northern India from around 2800 to 1900 BCE. A growing number of scholars believe that the culture reflected in the hymns of the *Rig-Veda*, the oldest of four Vedic hymnodies, is identical to or significantly overlaps with the Indus-Sarasvati civilization. My book *In Search of the Cradle of Civilization*, written with Subhash Kak and David Frawley, contains a review of the latest thinking on this important historical subject and chronicles the scholarly revolution that is under way. For a long time, it was thought that the Sanskrit-speaking Vedic people arrived in India no earlier than 1500 BCE and that they conquered the Dravidian-speaking natives as a result of their superior military power and skill. Upon discovery of the Indus-Sarasvati civilization—formerly called the Harappan or Indus civilization—in the early 1920s, scholars automatically assumed that invading Vedic Aryans were responsible for the destruction of that civilization. They simply moved the time of the invasion forward to around 1700 BCE.

The new evidence shows, however, that the Indus-Sarasvati civilization had undergone grave tribulations long before then. In particular, the great Sarasvati River, along which hundreds of villages and presumably also several large urban settlements were located, had ceased to exist by 1900 BCE. It is hard to imagine the human suffering caused by this tragedy, which was probably triggered by massive earthquakes and tectonic shifts. But the loss of what was once India's mightiest river did not spell the end of that civilization. Rather its center shifted from the Sarasvati River, whose dry bed now runs through the enormous Thar Desert, to the fertile banks of the Ganges. There a revival took place, which led to the familiar Hindu civilization, a direct offspring of the early Vedic civilization.

We can safely say that the earliest beginnings of the Yoga tradition can be found in the sacrificial ritualism of the Vedic people, who created both the impressive towns of the Indus and Sarasvati Rivers and also the beautiful and often enigmatic Vedic hymns. They practiced a spirituality that acknowledged the vital connection between the visible and the invisible realms. Through sacrificial rituals (*yajna*) they sought to establish, affirm, or strengthen the inner link with the heavenly powers, the gods and goddesses of the Vedic pantheon. The affairs of the world had to be conducted in the light of the divine order (*rita*) so that harmony, happiness, and prosperity could prevail.

In their quest for spiritual illumination, the Vedic Aryans fully understood that behind the multiplicity of worldly things, and behind the various deities, lies an irreducible unity, which they called the One (*eka*). The wise, declares one of the Rig-Vedic hymns (I.164.46), speak of it "in many ways"—a clear indication that they were no primitive polytheists but appreciated the language of relativity.

To reach that transcendental Singularity, the seer-bards, as another Rig-Vedic hymn (X.101.2) puts it, made their visions (*dhi*) harmonious and stretched them on the "loom" of cosmic existence. These inspired seers and hymn composers compared their sacred task to harnessing the plow (*yuga*)—a metaphor foreshadowing the later use of the term *yoga* to mean the harnessing or restraining of the senses and the mind so as to yield a quiet inner space. Tempted by the unruly senses, the mind, notes one Vedic bard, "flutters here and there like a bird" (*Rig-Veda* X.33.2). Only in the depth of the still heart can the liberating truth be found. For the heart is the seat of the Divine, the connecting point between the finite and the infinite. As the *Rig-Veda* states in mystical imagery:

> The whole universe is stationed in your home within the ocean, within the heart, in life. May we gain your honeyed wave that is brought to the edge, the junction of the waters. (IV.58.11)

The "honeyed wave" is the secret name of the butter used in the Vedic oblation, which is offered into the fire not only from a ladle but also from the human heart in the form of prayers, songs of praise, and inspired aspirations. The archaic Yoga of the Vedas often bore the name *tapas*, which literally means "heat" or "flow" and is a reference to the inner heat or energy produced by asceticism.

Thus Yoga looks back upon a history of five millennia and more. However, as a full-fledged spiritual tradition going by the name *yoga*, it is approximately two and a half millennia old. More specifically, the Yoga tradition crystallized at the time of the *Katha-Upanishad* (Secret Teaching of the Kathas), the *Bhagavad-Gita*, and the *Shvetashvatara-Upanishad* (Secret Teaching of the Whitest Horse). In the *Katha-Upanished*, Yama, God of Death, presents the Yoga tradition in the following way:

> Different indeed is the good (*shreyas*); different is the pleasant. Both to their various ends ensnare a person (*purusha*). Of these, it is well for one opting for the good. But he who chooses the pleasant falls short of the purpose [of life].
>
> The good and the pleasant have human [relevance]. Considering both, the sage distinguishes [them carefully]. The sage chooses the good over the pleasant. The fool, [intent on] acquiring and keeping (*yoga-kshema*), chooses the pleasant.
>
> After considering [this matter], you, O Naciketas, have rejected the pleasurable desires that appear pleasing. You have

not followed the way of wealth, in which many humans sink [as into a quagmire].

Ignorance (*avidya*) and what is known as wisdom (*vidya*) are far apart and divergent. I deem Naciketas to be desirous of wisdom, for many [lesser] desires have not distracted you.

Fools, abiding in the midst of ignorance and deeming themselves wise and learned, go about deluded, like blind men led by a blind man.

The passage (*samparaya*) [beyond death and to the ultimate Reality] is not evident to the fool, who is careless and deluded by the glamor of wealth. Thinking "this world exists, there is no other," he falls again into my [Death's] power.

Many are not even able to hear [of the ultimate Reality, the Self] and many do not know, though they have heard of It. Wondrous is the teacher, skillful he who has attained It! Wondrous the knower instructed by the skillful [teacher who knows the Self].

Taught by an inferior man, He [the ultimate Being] cannot be properly understood, being thought of as manifold. Being inconceivable and more minute in size than the most minute, there is no access to Him unless one is taught by another [who truly knows Him].

Not by reasoning is this understanding attainable but, dearest, [only] when taught by another for deep knowledge. You have obtained it, steadfast to truth. May we find, Naciketas, an inquirer like you. (I.2.1–9)

The youth named Naciketas is a symbol for all serious aspirants tired of earthly goods and desiring to know the glorious Reality, the ultimate Being. Yama, God of Death, is a symbol for the spiritual teacher (*guru*), who spells the end of the aspirant's self-centeredness and ordinary perception of the world. But just as death is merely a transformation from one level of existence to another, so the Lord of Death and all spiritual teachers after him are gateways to a new understanding and a new, sacred mode of life.

According to the anonymous author of the *Katha-Upanishad* (I.2.12), the wise individual leaves behind both joy and sorrow and realizes God (*deva*) in the cave of the heart through the agency of what is called *adhyatma-yoga*, the Yoga of the inmost self. This is the contemplation of the eternal Spirit, entailing the pacification of the mind and the senses. Yet, paradoxically, the Spirit or Self cannot be realized by effort alone. As the *Katha-Upanishad* (1.2.23) states, it can be attained "only by the one whom it chooses." In other words, there must be grace. The element of grace in the yogic process is emphasized by many other authorities, and it plays a leading role in Bhakti-Yoga, as first articulated in the *Bhagavad-Gita*.

This sacred text is the most treasured Yoga scripture in India; Mahatma Gandhi reverently called it "My Mother." It is embedded in the *Mahabharata* epic, one of India's two great national epics (the other is the *Ramayana*, whose spirituality falls in the category of asceticism, or *tapas*. The *Mahabharata* is the story of the war between two ancient Indian tribes, the Kurus and the Pandavas. Its legendary author Vyasa weaves all kinds of spiritual teachings into his lengthy description of the events leading up to the war, the eighteen-day war itself, and the aftermath. The *Bhagavad-Gita* is such a teaching episode, which occurs on the morning of the first battle when Arjuna, one of the Pandava princes, refuses to fight because he has spotted teachers and friends among the ranks of the enemy. Krishna, the divine incarnation serving as his charioteer, encourages him to do his duty as a warrior in this just war, whose purpose is to reestablish the lawful kingdom and moral order. The *Bhagavad-Gita* is the dialogue ensuing between them.

Yogic teachings also are given in the *Moksha-Dharma* (Liberation Teaching) section of the twelfth book of the *Mahabharata*. Like the teachings of the *Bhagavad-Gita*, they have been characterized as Epic Yoga or Preclassical Yoga and belong to varying periods extending from about 500 BCE to perhaps 100 CE. During this span of time, many Upanishads containing yogic teachings were composed. The

Shvetashvatara-Upanishad and the *Maitrayaniya-Upanishad* are especially significant.

The former work (I.3), whose curious name is apparently derived from the initiatory title of an unknown sage, speaks of the contemplative discipline (*dhyana-yoga*) by which the self-power of the hidden God is revealed. That God is called the Lord (*isha*) who supports the universe. The yogic discipline recommended involves meditative recitation of the sacred syllable OM—one of the most ancient practices of Yoga. Upon stilling the mind, the initiate may experience a number of internal visions. These are merely signposts and must not be confused with the ultimate goal of Self- or God-realization.

The yogic path is more systematically treated in the *Maitrayaniya-Upanishad*, which contains the following passage:

> This is the rule for accomplishing this [spiritual work]: breath control, sense-withdrawal, meditation, concentration, inquiry (*tarka*), and ecstasy (*samadhi*) are said to be Yoga. When seeing by means of this he sees the gold-colored maker, the Lord, the Spirit, the source of Brahma, then the sage, abandoning good and evil, makes everything unitary in the supreme Indestructible. For thus it has been said: "As birds and deer do not occupy a burning mountain, so the defects (*dosha*) never occupy a knower of the Absolute (*brahman*)." (IV.18)

Toward the end of this period in the evolution of Yoga or slightly later, perhaps around 200 CE, Classical Yoga emerged. It was codified by Patanjali in his famous *Yoga-Sutra* (Aphorisms of Yoga) and became the philosophical system of Yoga par excellence. Many Sanskrit commentaries have been written on this work, which consists of no more than 195 (or, in some editions, 196) terse aphorisms (*sutra*). The oldest and most valuable commentary, which is attributed to Vyasa (a name meaning "compiler"), is the *Yoga-Bhashya* (Speech on Yoga).

In addition to Classical Yoga, there were many other yogic schools in the period following Patanjali. Whereas Classical Yoga espoused a dualistic philosophy (distinguishing between spirit and matter), virtually all these other yogic schools subscribed to the nondualist (*advaita*) metaphysics that has been at home in India since ancient times. They are generally referred to as Postclassical Yoga.

These nondualist yogic teachings can be encountered, for instance, in the Puranas, encyclopedic compilations containing much religious and metaphysical information. Tradition speaks of eighteen major and as many minor Puranas, though their actual number is much higher, and each of these Sanskrit scriptures includes a more or less detailed treatment of the spiritual path. The best-known work of this genre is the *Bhagavata-Purana*, which contains the Krishna legends and much else besides. It was composed sometime in the tenth century CE. The name *purana* means "ancient" and points to the fact that the puranic heritage traces itself back to a very early age. A Purana is first mentioned in the *Atharva-Veda* (II.7.24), compiled some four thousand years ago, but the Puranic works known today are creations of a much later era.

A Purana-like tenth-century work is the beautifully imaginative and poetic *Yoga-Vasishtha*, comprising no fewer than 30,000 stanzas. This scripture promulgates nondualist Jnana-Yoga, which unfolds in seven stages. The highest stage of this Yoga is called *turya-ga* or "abiding in the Fourth," the Fourth being the transcendental Self beyond the three states of consciousness—waking, dream sleep, and deep sleep.

Another mine of yogic knowledge is the body of scriptures known as the Tantras (Webs), which belong to the tradition of Shaktism (or Shakti worship). They embody the esoteric teachings of Tantrism, about which more is said in chapter 11. The word *shakti* means "power" and refers to the spiritual energy—visualized as a goddess—behind the manifest universe. Tantrism is concerned with enlisting that goddess energy in the yogic process. Some traditional authorities identify 192 Tantras, of which the best known are the *Kula-Arnava-Tantra* (Tantra of the Kula Ocean) and the *Mahanirvana-Tantra* (Tantra of the Great Extinction). There are also numerous Buddhist Tantras, written in Sanskrit and Tibetan.

Yoga also is an integral part of Shaivism (Shiva worship), as given in the Agamas (Traditions), which are said to number twenty-eight in all, though over two hundred are known. Yogic teachings, moreover, are contained in the Samhitas (Compendiums) of Vaishnavism (Vishnu worship). Tradition recognizes 108 Samhitas, but one scholar has compiled a list of 215 and estimated that their original number was even higher. Thus Tantras, Agamas, and Samhitas form a vast literature that is relevant to the study of Yoga but has barely been researched.

A significant development within Yoga, emerging under the influence of Tantrism, is Hatha-Yoga (Forceful Yoga), which has its own scriptures. The creation of Hatha-Yoga is intimately connected with the name of the semilegendary adept Gorakshanatha (Hindi: Gorakhnath), who may have lived in the eleventh century CE. He is credited with the authorship of many Sanskrit texts, but these seem to have survived only as fragments and in quotations in later works. The most important Hatha-Yoga texts are the *Hatha-Yoga-Pradipika* (Light on the Forceful Yoga), the *Gheranda-Samhita* (Compendium of Gheranda), and the *Shiva-Samhita* (Shiva's Compendium). The first-mentioned work is the oldest, written sometime in the fourteenth century CE.

Besides the huge Sanskrit literature on Yoga, there are many Yoga texts in vernacular languages, notably Tamil. Particularly the poetic compositions of the South Indian Alvars (who were Vishnu worshipers) and the sixty-three Nayanmars (who were Shiva worshipers) must be mentioned. Their beautiful compositions, which speak of their heartfelt devotion to God and their longing to be united with Him, are a mainstay of South Indian Bhakti-Yoga. Perhaps the greatest Tamil work on Yoga is the *Tirumandiram* (Sacred Word) of Tirumular, who lived in the fifth or sixth century CE. The Tamil literature on Yoga has barely been studied, though it contains much important and fascinating information that complements the Sanskrit scriptures.

The history and literature of Yoga cut across many traditions within Hinduism. Various yogic approaches also can be found within the independent traditions of Buddhism and Jainism. In fact, the Buddha's "noble eightfold path" represents an early form of non-Vedic Yoga. There has been a lively osmosis between India's three great spiritual traditions and cultures—Hinduism, Buddhism, and Jainism. All this has created one of the most colorful and complex heritages on earth.

This overview has been little more than a rough thumbnail sketch. A detailed review of the history of Yoga and its literature can be found in my forthcoming book *The Yoga Tradition*.[1]

2

The Principal Branches of Yoga

There is nothing [on Earth] equal in purity to wisdom.
—BHAGAVAD-GITA IV.38

The Path of Wisdom: Jnana-Yoga

The yogic path outlined in the Upanishads mentioned in the previous chapter belongs to Jnana-Yoga, the spiritual discipline of wisdom (*jnana*). This is in fact the orientation typical of nearly all the more than two hundred known Upanishads, which are esoteric scriptures showing the way to self-understanding, self-transcendence, and mystical union. They praise wisdom as the supreme means of shattering all self-delusion and illusion, bringing the aspirant face to face with Reality, the Self, or Spirit. Wisdom is identification with the unitary essence of all objects. It is identification with the ultimate knower, or transcendental Subject, who is no different from the known. Wisdom is thus quite distinct from ordinary knowledge, which comes through the mediation of the senses, or through thought, and grasps the known from the outside.

Wisdom is a direct apprehension of Reality, or Self-realization. As such, wisdom has no informational content. It is simply truth-bearing, as the great Yoga adept Patanjali puts it in his *Yoga-Sutra* (I.48).

What is the truth that wisdom reveals? It is the truth, the reality, of the self-luminous Self, which is at once our innermost essence and the very foundation of the universe. In the words of Swami Vivekananda, a great nineteenth-century yogin and sage, who with great gusto represented Hinduism at the Parliament of Religions in 1894:

> Every particle in this body is continually changing; no one has the same body for many minutes together, and yet we think of it as the same body. So with the mind: one moment it is happy, another moment unhappy; one moment strong, another weak—an ever changing whirlpool. That cannot be the Spirit, which is infinite. . . . Any particle in this universe can change in relation to any other particle. But take the whole universe as one; then in relation to what can it move? There is nothing besides it. So this infinite Unit is unchangeable, immovable, absolute, and this is the Real Man.[1]

The Real Man, or the Real Woman, is the eternal gender-transcending Subject, the essential Self of all beings and things. This ultimate Unity cannot be sensed, experienced, or, strictly speaking, even known. However, it can be realized by going beyond all the mechanisms of sensing, experiencing, and knowing. In that case, it reveals itself to itself. It is by nature self-luminous. In other words, the Self shines forth as soon as we withdraw all our diverse mental projections from it; when we desist from identifying it as our body, our mind, or the external world. As Nisargadatta Maharaj, a contemporary master of Jnana-Yoga, put it:

> If you really find out what you are, you will see that you are not an individual, you are not a person, you are not a body. And people who cling to their body identity are not fit for this knowledge.[2]

Nisargadatta Maharaj continued:

> If you really want to understand this, you must give up your identification with the body. By all means, make use of the

body, but don't consider yourself to be the body while acting in this world. Identify yourself with the consciousness, which dwells in the body. . . . So long as you identify yourself as the body, your experience of pain and sorrow will increase day by day. That is why you must give up this identification, and you should take yourself as the consciousness. . . . When the body falls, the principle which always remains is You. If you identify yourself with the body, you will feel that you are dying, but in reality there is no death because you are not the body. Let the body be there or not be there, your existence is always there; it is eternal.[3]

Ramana Maharshi, a Self-realized master, wrote:

Enquiring "Who am I?" within the mind, and reading the heart, the "I" collapses. Instantly the real "I" appears (as "I," "I"), which, although it manifests itself as "I" is not the ego, but the true being.[4]

Jnana-Yoga thus consists in a radical dismantling of all our delusions and illusions, attachments, fears, sorrows, opinions, desires, hopes, and expectations. Every experience or piece of information is approached with the insight that this does not represent the Truth, the Self—"not thus, not thus" (*neti neti*), as Sage Yajnavalkya put it long ago.[5] This *via negativa* is the path most characteristic of the Vedanta tradition, which avows a nondualist metaphysics: "There is only the One; all else is illusory." Everything that is not the Self is illusion (*maya*), which is compared to a dream in the Yoga and Vedanta scriptures. Self-realization, or enlightenment, is our awakening from that dream.

This approach calls for sustained keen discernment (*viveka*) between the Real and the unreal, followed by an equally demanding and uncompromising attitude of dispassion (*vairagya*) toward everything that stands exposed as being other than the eternal Self. After all, we might know that something is not good for us but continue to indulge in it. Dispassion or nonattachment is one of the keystones of spiritual life. Without it there can be no real inner growth. Hence since time immemorial, the practitioners of Yoga have cultivated the ideal of renunciation (*samnyasa*). Some have interpreted this to mean abandoning worldly life in favor of voluntary simplicity in the secluded environment of a hermitage or even a life of perpetual homelessness and wandering. Others, however, have taken renunciation to be primarily an inner attitude, which may or may not be accompanied by outward abstention. For the practitioner of Jnana-Yoga, who is called a *jnana-yogin* or *jnanin*, renunciation comes naturally as a result of his or her deep understanding of the pattern of life and the true nature of reality.

The Path of Selfless Action: Karma-Yoga

Though growing out of the earlier Vedic heritage, the teachings of the Upanishads were a novel development in the evolution of Hinduism. Whereas the Vedic spirituality revolved around the ideal of sacrifice *combined with* meditation, the Upanishads preached the inner sacrifice *of* meditation. Traditionally, this distinction was couched in terms of wisdom (*jnana*) versus action (*karman*), meaning primarily ritual action.

A growing number of people were attracted to the life of wisdom and renunciation as espoused by the Upanishadic sages, so much so that, around the middle of the first millennium BCE, some authorities began to oppose this widespread movement. They argued that a person should wait until all the duties of a householder had been fulfilled and the children were fully grown before retiring to the forest or mountain solitude. Their reasoning was that all too often the call to renunciation led to abandoned families and unmet social obligations. The lawgivers favored a lifestyle ideally unfolding in four stages (*ashrama*)—those of the student, the householder, the forest-dweller (in late maturity), and the freely wandering ascetic (in old age). In this way, the practitioner gave active life its proper due before taking up the contemplative lifestyle of a renouncer (*samnyasin*), who is wholly dedicated to the pursuit of truth through solitary meditation, introspection, and wisdom.

In the middle of the first millennium BCE, a first powerful effort was made to integrate wisdom with action in the teaching of the *Bhagavad-Gita*. This effort also brought the strong human capacity for love (*bhakti*) into the equation. In fact, this venerated scripture stands at the threshold of an entire long-lived spiritual movement of devotionalism, focusing on the worship of God in personal form, notably Lord Krishna. This movement is known as the way of love or *bhakti-marga*, which is explained in the next section.

While love or devotion is central to Krishna's message, his teaching is unthinkable without the corollaries of wisdom and selfless action. In Krishna's understanding, the Yoga of action consists in the execution of one's allotted work in the proper fashion without any thought of personal gain or self-aggrandizement, or even praise. As he put it:

> Not by abstention from actions does a man enjoy action-transcendence, nor by renunciation alone does he approach perfection.
>
> For, not even for a moment can anyone ever remain without performing action. Everyone is unwittingly made to act by the qualities (*guna*) issuing from Nature.
>
> He who restrains his organs of action but sits remembering in his mind the objects of the senses is called a self-bewildered hypocrite.
>
> So—more excellent is he, O Arjuna, who, controlling the senses with his mind, embarks unattached on Karma-Yoga with his organs of action.
>
> You must do the allotted action, for action is superior to inaction; not even your body's processes can be accomplished by inaction.

This world is action-bound, save when this action is [intended] as sacrifice. With that purpose, O son of Kunti, engage in action devoid of attachment. (III.4–9)

Therefore always perform unattached the proper deed, for the man who performs action without attachment attains the Supreme. (III.19)

Krishna's Karma-Yoga has sometimes been wrongly used to justify any military action. However, it must be remembered that the war fought by Arjuna and his four brothers against the Kurus had the specific purpose of restoring the moral order (*dharma*). This alone explains Lord Krishna's intervention. As a divine incarnation, he is born whenever the moral order has collapsed and the world is enveloped in spiritual darkness.

The follower of Karma-Yoga, who is known as a *karma-yogin*, acts in daily life so as to lessen lawlessness (*adharma*) and increase virtue (*dharma*) or harmony. Like Mahatma Gandhi, Vinoba Bhave, or Mother Teresa, he or she works for the welfare of others. As a true yogic discipline, Karma-Yoga seeks to overcome the ego-personality with its egotistic desires and attitudes, carelessness, doubts, and fears. This approach is often portrayed as an easy option, but in fact it calls for great discernment. As Krishna said:

What is action? What is inaction? Herein even the seer-poets (*kavi*) are bewildered. I shall declare to you that action which, when understood, will set you free from ill.

Indeed, [the *yogin*] ought to understand [the nature] of action, he ought to understand misaction (*vikarman*), and he ought to understand inaction. Impenetrable is the way of action.

He who sees inaction in action and action in inaction is wise among men, yoked, performing whole actions. (IV.16–18)

Whole (*kritsna*) actions are those that are guided by wisdom and are free from attachment and also otherwise appropriate. Then action cannot defile a person, cannot create a karmic debt. For this kind of action to become possible, a person must first be whole himself or herself. At the same time, Karma-Yoga is a path to this inner wholeness.

The Path of Love-Devotion: Bhakti-Yoga

A reverential and devotional attitude in spiritual life was cultivated already by the seer-bards of Vedic times. However, as an independent path, Bhakti-Yoga emerged only around the middle of the first millennium BCE, primarily in connection with the theistic religions centering on the worship of Krishna (a devine incarnation of Vishnu) and Rudra or Shiva. The religious tradition that has Krishna as its focal point was first given expression in the beautiful verses of the *Bhagavad-Gita*. In the same era, the Shiva worshipers created the *Shvetashvatara-Upanishad*, which contains the following declaration:

> The God who is in fire, who is in water, who has entered the whole world, who is in plants, who is in trees—to that God be adoration, adoration. (II.17)

The wise composer of this Upanishad next divulges his own spiritual attainment, which lends authority to his words:

> I know this great Person (*purusha*),
> sun-colored, beyond darkness.
> Only by knowing Him does one go beyond death.
> There is no other path for going [to Him].
>
> Nothing is higher than He,
> nothing is smaller than He, nothing greater.
> The One stands like a tree established in Heaven.
> By Him, the [supreme] Person, this whole [universe] is filled.
>
> That which is beyond this [world]
> is formless, free from ill.
> Those who know That become immortal,
> but others encounter only suffering. (III.8–10)

In the *Bhagavad-Gita*, it is the Lord himself who speaks, disclosing the secrets of Bhakti-Yoga:

> [He] Whose self is yoked in Yoga and who everywhere beholds the same, sees the Self abiding in all beings and all beings in the Self.
>
> He who sees Me everywhere and sees all in Me, to him I am not lost, nor is he [ever] lost to Me.
>
> He who is intent on oneness *(ekatva)* and loves Me, abiding in all beings in whatever [state] he exists, that *yogin* dwells in Me. (VI.29–32)

The path of Bhakti-Yoga is constant remembrance of the Divine, whether it is known as Krishna, Rama, Mahadeva, Radha, Sita, or Parvati, or by some other name of God or Goddess. This remembrance can take many forms—from rituals dedicated to the Divine to love-intoxicated chanting, singing, and dancing, to deeply felt attunement in meditation and ecstatic absorption into the Divine. The practitioner of this yogic path, who is called a *bhakta* (devotee), may look upon the Divine as one might look upon a parent, a friend, or a lover. In every case, however, he or she seeks to cultivate true intimacy with God or Goddess until mystical union is achieved. "The essence of Bhakti-Yoga," wrote the Indian scholar Inder Pal Sachdev, "lies in complete unconditional self-surrender to the Highest Being."[6] Surendra Nath Dasgupta, one of the great savants of modern India, described the devotee as follows:

> So great is his passion for God that it consumes all his earthly passions. . . . The bhakta who is filled with such a passion does not experience it merely as an undercurrent of joy which waters the depths of his heart in his own privacy, but as a torrent that overflows the caverns of his heart into all his senses. Through all his senses he realizes it as if it were a sensuous delight; with his heart and soul he feels it as a spiritual intoxication of joy. Such a person is beside himself with

this love of God. He sings, laughs, dances and weeps. He is no longer a person of this world.[7]

This passionate love for the Divine was alive in male saints like Prahlada, Vallabha, Caitanya, Ramanuja, Namm Alvar, Namdeva, Kabir, Nanak, and Tukaram, as well as female mystics like Andal and Mirabai.

Unlike the *jnana-yogins*, the followers of Bhakti-Yoga often prefer a dualist metaphysics over a strictly nondualist philosophy. Some schools of this branch of Yoga even deny that perfect merging or identification with the Lord can ever be achieved, postulating an unbridgeable gap between Creator and creation. Yet even these schools enthusiastically promote the pursuit of mystical union, however incomplete. For, as they insist, only in communion with the Divine can lasting happiness be found.

The Path of Sacred Sound: Mantra-Yoga

We do not know when the consciousness-altering effects of sound were discovered, but rhythmic drumming and chanting undoubtedly belong to the earliest cultural heritage of humanity. It is an integral part of shamanism, which preceded the Yoga tradition and contributed many elements to it. Already in Vedic times, the seers and sages considered sound a transformative vehicle, and they regarded the hymns as being charged with numinous power. Thus recitation and chanting were early on cultivated as potent means of focusing the mind, pacifying the senses, and elevating consciousness to a higher level of functioning, creating the proper conditions for a deep spiritual opening.

As one hymn of the *Rig-Veda* (X.71.3) states, "through sacrifice they walked on the path of Vac and found it in the seers." Vac is divine speech, the immortal sound revealed to the seers of ancient times. "Many who have eyes," declares the next verse, "have not seen Vac; many who have ears do not hear her." The divine Word, which is heard and followed by all the deities, is manifested in the seer's ecstatic vision (*dhi*) and proclaimed in his inspired hymns. In the *Atharva-Veda* (XIX.9.3), Vac is called the "supreme Goddess, strengthened by prayer (*brahman*)."[8] It is Vac, the imperishable Word, that the Vedic seers sought to track down. The Word that is imperishable (*akshara*) was a great secret in ancient times but later—as early as the *Yajur-Veda*—was disclosed as the immortal sound OM—the first of all *mantras* or numinous sounds.

The *Yajur-Veda* also contains other similar mantric sounds, notably HIM, HUM, SVAHA, and VASHAT. These were interjected at various stages of the sacrificial rituals, but none ever gained the same prominence as the sacred syllable OM, symbol of the Absolute.

Out of this ritualistic use of certain sounds grew, in due course, the yogic practice of recitation known as *japa* in which a *mantra* is repeated over and over again to calm the mind. Often the *mantras* used in this way are the names of particular deities, such as Shiva or Rama. The Transcendental Meditation (TM) movement is based on the mental sounding of certain *mantras*. The meditative recitation of *mantras* is often done in conjunction with a rosary (*mala*), usually consisting of 108 beads.

Mantra-Yoga came into its own with the rise of Tantrism nearly two thousand years ago. Subsequently it developed into an independent yogic approach, containing many ritualistic elements. This full-fledged system is outlined in such Sanskrit works as the *Mantra-Yoga-Samhita* (Compendium of Mantra-Yoga) and the encyclopedic *Mantra-Mahodadhi* (Ocean of Mantras). This yogic approach is discussed in more detail in chapter 9.

The Royal Path of Raja-Yoga

Raja-Yoga is synonymous with Classical Yoga, as formulated by Patanjali in his *Yoga-Sutra* around two thousand years ago. This school is traditionally considered one of the six orthodox systems of

Hindu philosophy. Although Classical Yoga was influential, it did not survive as a school of yogic practice in its own right. Its decline was largely due to its dualist metaphysics in an overwhelmingly nondualist philosophical climate, shaped by the powerful tradition of Vedanta. However, its model of the yogic path was adopted by many other schools. As the renowned historian of religion Mircea Eliade observed, "It is from this system that one must start in order to understand the position of yoga in the history of Indian thought."[9] It also is this school of thought that provides the most systematic access to the practical dimension of Yoga. Hence a careful study of the *Yoga-Sutra* can be heartily recommended to all Western Yoga enthusiasts.

Patanjali, to whom the *Yoga-Sutra* is attributed and about whom nothing is known, offered many helpful definitions of the various aspects of Yoga, notably its eight principal limbs (*anga*):

1. Moral restraint (*yama*), comprising nonharming (*ahimsa*), truthfulness (*satya*), nonstealing (*asteya*), chastity (*brahmacarya*), and greedlessness (*aparigraha*)
2. Discipline (*niyama*), consisting of purity (*shauca*), contentment (*samtosha*), asceticism (*tapas*), study (*svadhyaya*), and devotion to the Lord (*ishvara-pranidhana*)
3. Posture (*asana*)
4. Breath control (*pranayama*)
5. Sense withdrawal (*pratyahara*)
6. Concentration (*dharana*)
7. Meditation (*dhyana*)
8. Ecstasy (*samadhi*)

These practices are discussed in later chapters of this book. Here I simply wish to mention that moral restraint is the foundation of the other limbs and must be observed at all times. Only then can the path of progressive unification and simplification succeed and lead to the various ecstatic states of consciousness and, ultimately, to liberation or Self-realization.

The Path of Inner Power: Hatha-Yoga

The word *hatha* means "force" or "forceful" and refers to that branch of Yoga that attempts self-transformation and self-transcendence by the arduous means of physical purification and strengthening. The idea behind Hatha-Yoga is that a frail or diseased body can prove a serious obstacle on the path to liberation and that therefore the body must be properly trained. This training is particularly important in Hatha-Yoga because at the core of this spiritual discipline is a potentially dangerous process known as the awakening of the *kundalini-shakti*. This is the arousal of the power of consciousness in the lowest psychospiritual center (*cakra*) of the body and its conduction to the highest center at the crown of the head. If the body is not properly prepared, the awakened *kundalini* can cause tremendous physical and mental problems. As the texts declare, the *kundalini* can lead either to liberation or to bondage. We might say that it can lead either to heaven or to hell, depending on the purity of the pathways through which the *kundalini-shakti*, or serpent power, must flow to reach the topmost psychospiritual center.

Hatha-Yoga consequently incorporates in its program a great many techniques for physical cleansing and stabilization of the body's energies. It also includes many postures (*asana*), which are used to maintain or restore the *yogin*'s well-being, to improve the body's flexibility and vitality, and also, in some cases, to serve as suitable postures for prolonged meditation. The heart of Hatha-Yoga is unquestionably breath control (*pranayama*), and a variety of techniques are given to manipulate the body's energy (*prana*) via the breath.

This is the form of Yoga best known in the West, though its deeper spiritual and philosophical foundations are rarely understood. It is widely reduced to gymnastics and fitness training, without any reference to, or experience of, the *kundalini* and higher states of consciousness, never mind the great ideal of spiritual liberation. Traditionally, however, Hatha-Yoga has always been looked upon as a ladder to Raja-Yoga, that is, to Self-realization through meditation and ecstasy. The contemporary Hatha-Yoga master B. K. S. Iyengar, who has trained the majority of American Hatha-Yoga teachers, made this pertinent remark: "The original idea of yoga is freedom and beatitude, and the by-products which come along the way, including physical health, are secondary for the practitioner."[10]

Historically speaking, Hatha-Yoga is unthinkable without the prior development of Tantrism or Tantra-Yoga. For the awakening of the *kundalini-shakti*, which is the goal of Hatha-Yoga, was central to Tantric esotericism long before the emergence of Hatha-Yoga. In some ways, Hatha-Yoga is an offshoot of Tantrism, and many of its ritualistic elements are adaptations from the Tantric heritage. The ultimate purpose of Tantra-Yoga is to bring about the reunion of the polarized energy and consciousness, the merging of God Shiva and Goddess Shakti, which yields the blissful nectar of immortality in ecstasy. The Tantric path is outlined more fully in chapter 11.

3

The Teacher, the Disciple, and the Path

The knowers who have seen the Truth will instruct you in wisdom.
—BHAGAVAD-GITA IV.34

Heart Knowledge beyond Intellectual Learning

Even if we read a thousand books on oceanography or on maritime adventures, we cannot really understand the ocean unless we jump into the water ourselves and get wet. Then we can feel its power and learn to both respect and trust it. The situation is similar in regard to the ocean of Yoga (*yoga-arnava*). We can learn many facts about Yoga, but they will give us only an external view of it. In order to truly understand Yoga, we must engage its living reality and allow it to teach us.

The experiential nature of Yoga has always been emphasized by its advocates. Thus Vyasa quotes in his *Yoga-Bhashya* (Speech on Yoga), the earliest available Sanskrit commentary on Patanjali's *Yoga-Sutra* (Aphorisms of Yoga), an ancient saying:

> Yoga must be known through Yoga. Yoga grows through Yoga.
> He who is attentive toward Yoga long delights in Yoga. (III.6)

Many centuries earlier, the *Mahabharata* epic expressed the same idea in these words:

> He who does not know the meaning of a book carries only a burden; but he who knows the reality behind a book's meaning, for him the teaching of that book is not in vain. (XII.293.25)

The Yoga tradition has a large and diversified literature to which Western Yoga enthusiasts have added a huge volume of books. So long as the knowledge communicated in those books is not translated into practical experience, it remains barren. Mere intellectual knowledge is not adequately transformative.

Hence the *Yoga-Shikha-Upanishad* (Secret Doctrine of the Crest of Yoga), a medieval Sanskrit work, warns of the "snare of textbooks" (*shastra-jala*), referring to bookish learning without accompanying experience. Similarly, in the *Kula-Arnava-Tantra* (Family Ocean Tantra), God Shiva says to his divine spouse:

> O Beloved, creatures (*pashu*) who have fallen into the deep well of the six systems [of philosophy] do not know the ultimate purpose [of life] and remain constrained by the bond of creatures.
>
> Struggling in the terrifying ocean of the *Vedas* and textbooks, they stay [trapped] in the waves of time [as if] possessed by a demon, chanting "whither?" (I.87–88)

In a subsequent verse, Shiva complains about those who know much but have not actually tasted the food, by which he means the nourishment of the spirit. Thus while scriptural authority is held high in Yoga, it is not placed above personal experience and spiritual realization. The pivot of all Yoga is direct apprehension (*pratyaksha*) of the truth through personal spiritual practice. This is captured in the following words of the *Yoga-Bhashya*:

> Through study (*svadhyaya*) he should cultivate Yoga;
> through Yoga he should cultivate study; through the con-
> junction of study and Yoga the supreme Self manifests.
> (I.28)

Vyasa's advice to give both knowledge and experience their due
weight reflects the ever-present concern of the *yogin* to practice balance. Practice that is not supported by a solid understanding of the
Yoga tradition is apt to produce self-delusion. On the other hand,
study that is not anchored in practice is likely to lead to a false sense
of accomplishment without yielding any spiritual gain. In the final
analysis, however, Yoga puts the heart above the head, experience
above thought.

Hence, since the earliest times, the Yoga scriptures and authorities
have always stressed the necessity for guidance. Only someone who
has traveled the road will know its pitfalls and can help prevent those
who follow in his or her footsteps from falling into obvious and not-
so-obvious traps.

The Guru: He Whose Counsel Is Weighty

The Sanskrit language has many words for "teacher," but only the
designation *guru* captures the essential function of the teacher who
serves others as a spiritual guide. The word means "heavy" or
"weighty" and refers to someone whose counsel is significant. According to an esoteric etymology, *guru* is divided into its two syllables, *gu* and *ru*, which respectively are said to stand for "darkness"
and "dispeller." Thus the *guru* is a teacher who is capable of removing the student's spiritual darkness, or blindness.

Often such a teacher is called a *sad-guru*, which can mean both a
"true teacher" and a "teacher of the Truth." The term *sat* (which for
euphonic reasons is changed to *sad* when followed by a soft conso-
nant or vowel) can be used either as an adjective or as a noun. In the

latter sense, it generally connotes the ultimate Reality, or Truth. As Ramana Maharshi explained:

> The Guru is one who at all times abides in the profound depths of the Self. He never sees any difference between himself and others and is quite free from the idea that he is the Enlightened or the Liberated One, while those around him are in bondage or the darkness of ignorance. . . . There is no difference between God, Guru, and the Self.[1]

The *sad-guru* is, above all, a spiritual presence. As such he (or she) is a great power that can prove transformative for those who are open to its influence. Hence the traditional authorities all recommend that earnest seekers seek out the company of such beings as much as possible. The practice of sitting at the feet of great, enlightened masters is known as *sat-sanga*, or "contact with Reality."

The Sanskrit scriptures acknowledge that a *sad-guru* is a rarity among teachers. As the *Kula-Arnava-Tantra* puts it:

> O Devi, there are many *gurus* here on Earth who give what is other than the Self, but hard to find in all the worlds is the *guru* who reveals the Self. (XIII.106)

Many *gurus* have pilgrimaged only part of the way to Truth, or Reality, but are still in a position to guide an aspirant to their own level of attainment. Other teachers know how to repeat the teachings but have no experiential knowledge themselves and thus are unreliable and even dangerous guides. Finally, there are those who—as the texts admit—are simply fakes. To cite the *Kula-Arnava-Tantra* again:

> Many are the *gurus* who rob a disciple of his wealth, but rare is the *guru* who removes a disciple's [spiritual] afflictions. (XIII.108)

A student would therefore do well to ascertain to which category a teacher belongs before committing to long-term pupilage. Sadly, this warning ought to be particularly heeded by Western students of Yoga, for the marketplace is swamped with would-be teachers. There is some protection in a student's own purity of intent, and of course we often learn through our more painful experiences. Fortunately, even today there are *sad-gurus* who can pass on the ancient wisdom of Yoga, but they are seldom those teachers who are in the limelight or clamoring for disciples. A *sad-guru* very likely will test aspirants, perhaps by showing indifference toward them or even by first outright rejecting them. Only those who are truly committed to the spiritual path, who yearn for guidance, and who also have a certain degree of maturity and self-understanding will not be put off by the *sad-guru*'s behavior and stay on. And then the real trials and work of self-transformation begin.

Discipleship can flourish only when the aspirant brings the utmost dedication and intelligence to it. Intelligence, in the sense of fine discernment, is necessary not only to follow the *guru*'s instructions properly but also to constantly see the *guru* not merely as another individual but as a *function*—namely the function of countering the egoistic tendencies in the disciple. Without adequate discernment, disciples all too easily get caught up in personality conflicts and projections, which undermine the spiritual process set in motion by the *guru*. As the *Kula-Arnava-Tantra* states:

> The *guru* must not be considered a [mere] mortal. If he is so considered, then one will have no success at all from *mantras* or the worship of deities. (XII.46)

The Disciple

Discipleship (*shishyata*), which is an integral aspect of all spiritual traditions, has a long history. Unfortunately, it has been eroded by modern secularism, with its emphasis on intellectual learning and the communication of information rather than education in wisdom through lived experience. Because of this modern mind-set, few Western seekers are able to relate rightly either to the Yoga tradition or to its *gurus*. All too often they approach spiritual teachers with wrong expectations and faulty attitudes. They frequently fail to understand that discipleship is a sacred contract between *guru* and pupil, involving unusual commitments and obligations for both parties. I have addressed this issue in depth in my book *Holy Madness*.[2]

Here is how the Yoga tradition characterizes a fully qualified disciple (*shishya; cela* in Hindi):

> Endowed with great energy and enthusiasm, intelligent, heroic, learned in the scriptures, having the inclination to practice, free from delusion, unconcerned, . . . eating moderately, with senses under control, fearless, pure, skillful, giving, and a shelter for all people. (*Shiva-Samhita* V.26–30)

Exceedingly few aspirants can claim to possess these virtuous qualities! Most bring far less to the demands of discipleship. This has always been so, and the great teachers have shown tremendous compassion and tolerance toward their disciples. The desire to grow spiritually generally precedes the aspirant's initial capacity to engage the spiritual path with unwavering certainty and energy. The *Mahabharata* declares:

> The great path is difficult and those who tread it successfully to the end are not many. But he is called someone of great fault (*baha-dosha*) who, having set out on it, ceases to continue and turns back. (V.52)

But, as the *Bhagavad-Gita* (II.40) reminds us, no effort made on the spiritual path is ever lost. Particularly Western students, who live in an environment that tends to be unsupportive of our highest spiritual aspirations, must remember this piece of wisdom, for they may experience many false starts or temporary setbacks on the path. But even in the most ideal of circumstances Yoga is never easy, because it demands a complete self-transformation: From an ego-personality wrapped up in personal concerns and habit patterns, the aspirant must become a self-transcending being whose attention is freed from selfish interests and capable of contemplating the transcendental Self and hearing the plight of others.

Spiritual discipleship aims at the dissolution of the thing called "disciple." Its success is measured by the degree to which the aspirant is transformed from a self-involved seeker hankering after enlightenment, guruship, or power into a being filled with wisdom, compassion, patience, generosity, and all the other great virtues praised in the spiritual traditions of the world.

Initiation, Spiritual Transmission, and the Lineage

Yoga is a full-fledged initiatory tradition. Initiation, as the American philosopher Dane Rudhyar astutely observed, always "implies a reordering of energies and purposes."[3] Thus initiation represents, as he put it, "a victory over the inertia of habits of thinking-feeling and behaving in terms of what was once normal functioning, a dying to the past and rebirth to an unfamiliar and uncertain future—thus a victory over fear and an act of faith in the yet-unknown."[4]

Initiation involves a definite shift in the aspirant's inner world. It marks a most significant transition—from a secular to a sacred way of life. Henceforth he or she is placed in a mighty stream of intent and energy that, if the aspirant cooperates sufficiently, will sooner or later conduct him or her to the desired goal of liberation. The *Kula-Arnava-Tantra* states:

> There can be no liberation without initiation. Thus it has been said in the *Shiva-Shasana*. And there can be no such

[initiation] without a lineage from one teacher to the next teacher. (XIV.3)

Lineage (*parampara*) is very important in Yoga, as it is in many other traditions. One can compare it to a powerful electrical cable running from the present teacher to all previous teachers, whether embodied or dwelling in the invisible realms. Through initiation (*diksha*), the aspirant is adopted into a particular lineage and thereby becomes heir to its current of spiritual realization and potency. This increases his or her likelihood of making safe and rapid progress on the spiritual path. Initiation has often been compared to a second birth, and it is a powerful rite of passage.

Diksha is a form of spiritual empowerment. Usharbudh Arya, a meditation teacher living in the United States, notes that initiation "may be regarded as a spiritual sacrament confined to no particular religion." He goes on to say:

> The initiation begins the process of sanctifying the initiate by placing in his mind a seed that might grow over a period of time if irrigated and nourished through regular practice and related disciplines. . . . It is a process of direct transfer of mental energy from one mind to another.[5]

The scriptures distinguish various types of initiation, depending on the context in which it occurs. It can be formal or informal, gradual or sudden, associated with all kinds of external rituals, internal meditations, and visualization or completely independent of any effort on the part of the disciple. A *guru* may simply gaze into the disciple's eyes and transmit his or her own realization, which then results in an immediate change in the disciple's consciousness. Swami Muktananda initiated thousands of Westerners in this way, which is known as *shambhavi-diksha*. The word *shambhavi* is the adjectival form of *shambhu* ("benevolent"), which is an epithet of God Shiva. The name is meant to indicate that this type of initiation is a direct transmission of divine energy (*shakti*).

All initiations, in varying degrees, augment consciousness or awareness and energy in the disciple, thereby empowering him or her to put the teacher's instructions more effectively into practice and also to develop an attitude of dispassion.

Another Sanskrit term for initiation is *abhisheka*, which means literally "sprinkling"—a form of spiritual water baptism. What is sprinkled on the aspirant is the *guru*'s blessings.

The Discipline of Self-Transcendence

Yoga, explained Patanjali, is powered by both practice and dispassion. Practice (*abhyasa*) is the discipline of inner unification or simplification by which the clutter of external things and concerns is held at bay and which discloses the ultimate simplicity, or singularity, of the transcendental Self (*purusha*). As Patanjali noted, for practice to be successful it must be steady and cultivated over a long stretch of time. In his *Yoga-Bhashya* (I.13), Vyasa defines practice as "an endeavor (*prayatna*) with the purpose [of achieving an undisturbed flow of consciousness], a dynamic application (*virya*), or an effort (*utsaha*)." In other words, practice refers to the yogic struggle to conquer the ordinary mind, which is habitually agitated and removed from the realization of peace and tranquillity.

Dispassion (*vairagya*), according to the *Yoga-Sutra* (I.15) of Patanjali, is "the awareness of mastery of him who is not thirsting after visible [that is, earthly] and revealed [that is, invisible] things." The "revealed" objects spoken of here are those promised in the sacred texts, such as heavenly delights. The goal of Yoga is not any celestial domain but the transcendental Reality, or Spirit, which exists beyond all realms of manifestation, including the heavenly worlds of the Hindu religion.

While practice opens up higher experiences of the subtle or "invisible" realms, the *yogin* knows these to be only of relative value and pushes on toward the nonlocal reality of the Self. In this the *yogin* is guided by a growing mood of dispassion, which helps in renouncing even the greatest pleasures to be harvested in the most subtle realms of existence. For the *yogin* knows that lasting happiness comes only with Self-realization. The bliss arising from Self-realization is not dependent on any object but is innate to the Self and therefore can never be lost, or even decreased or increased.

Adepts express their inner dispassion in various ways. Some may spontaneously abandon all societal contact and live naked in a remote cave. Others, equally spontaneously, may immerse themselves in social activity for the benefit of others, without the slightest attachment to success, failure, or fame. They become the true masters of Karma-Yoga. The Indian tradition knows of great kings, such as Rama and Janaka, who lived from this enlightened point of view. Yet other adepts enjoying perfect dispassion may adopt a mendicant life, wandering from village to village to bless people, bring hope and spiritual light to them, and ease their burdens. All these adepts follow perfectly their inner law (*sva-dharma*), living out their human lives in a state of perpetual grace. Whether they are active in the world or have withdrawn from it, they unfailingly radiate peace to all, thereby spiritually uplifting humanity and all other beings on this planet.

4

Happiness and the Moral Foundations of Yoga

One should lift oneself up by the Self.[1]
—Bhagavad-Gita VI.5

"Follow Your Bliss"

When asked how best to live, the American mythologist Joseph Campbell responded, "Follow your bliss." But what is a person's bliss? Campbell, who was well acquainted with India's religious traditions, did not mean "Follow your pleasure." He also knew full well that bliss, or *ananda*, is no one person's property but the essential quality of the transcendental Reality itself. Thus his advice implies a dedication to authentic Selfhood (*atmata*) rather than the ego-personality (*ahamkara*), which, metaphysically speaking, is a false center of experience.

The domain of the ego-personality is the finite world, which, because of its finitude, is a source of unending suffering (*duhkha*). For even in our experiences of pleasure we can detect an element of pain, if only we dare look closely enough. At least this is the viewpoint of the sages of ancient and modern India, who have understood that the very fact that even our most exquisite pleasures do not last is a painful insight. Also, they realized that if it were possible to prolong any pleasurable experience enough, it would be attended by boredom, which is a form of suffering.

As Gautama, the founder of Buddhism, observed after profound meditation:

> This, monks, is the noble truth of suffering: Birth is sorrowful; old age is sorrowful; illness is sorrowful; death is sorrowful; grief, distress, and despair are sorrowful; to be united with what is unwanted is sorrowful; to be separated from what is wanted is sorrowful; not to obtain what is desired is sorrowful; in short, the five "groups" are sorrowful. (*Mahavagga* I.6.19)

The five groups (*skandha*) are the body, sensations, perceptions, thoughts, and consciousness. These are inherently impermanent and therefore not conducive to true happiness or bliss.

Bliss belongs to the unconditional Reality beyond body, mind, and the world of finite objects. It is this bliss that has always been the aspiration of the great seekers and that those who have transcended the ego-personality realize as their own innermost nature. In the archaic *Taittiriya-Upanishad* (Secret Doctrine of the Taittiriyas) we read:

> Let there be a youth, a good youth, well read, quick, firm, and strong. Let this whole earth be replete with wealth for him. That is one human bliss.
>
> A hundred human blisses are one bliss of the human spirits—also of a learned man who is not afflicted with desire. (II.8)

The text then compares the bliss of the human spirits to the hundredfold more intense bliss of the divine spirits, to the ten thousand times more intense bliss of the ancestors, and so on, past the lower deities and higher deities all the way to the bliss of the Absolute (*brahman*), which is reckoned to be one hundred quintillion times more blissful than ordinary human bliss. This is a figure containing twenty zeros.

What this intriguing passage seeks to convey is that the bliss realized by a person who is free from the stranglehold of desire exceeds all possible forms of bliss that can be experienced in the human and divine realms. As we ascend the ladder of existence to the highest divine realm of the Creator, we experience greater and greater joy. But nothing compares to the delight that is essential to the transcendental Self, which is the Absolute (*brahman*), the very foundation of existence. "This is [a person's] highest path," declared Yajnavalkya in the *Brihad-Aranyaka-Upanishad* (IV.3.32). "This is his highest accomplishment. This is his highest world. This is his highest bliss. Other beings live on a mere fraction of that bliss." Therefore the sages have always asked: Why settle for less than that? This is also the orientation in the Yoga tradition.

The Great Vow of Moral Discipline

In order to gain the unsurpassable bliss of the Self, the *yogin* willingly adopts a life of strict discipline. The aspirant begins by carefully regulating his or her moral behavior. This forms the bedrock of all types of Yoga. Reduced to its bare bones, yogic morality is the recognition of the universal Self in all other beings. The various moral rules expounded in the Yoga scriptures are a symbolic bow to the Self within the other person. Thus Yoga morality is inseparable from Yoga metaphysics. In their moral conduct, the *yogins* aspire to preserve the moral order of the cosmos within the limited orbit of their personal existence. In other words, they seek to uphold the ideals of harmony and balance. This endeavor is by no means unique to Yoga. Rather the moral code followed by its practitioners is universal and can be found in all the great religious traditions of the world.

As the American social critic Theodore Roszak correctly understood, the *yogin's* first step must necessarily be a moral one:

[H]igher consciousness is born out of conscience. "Consciousness"/"conscience": the very words are related, reminding us that we cannot expect to expand spiritual awareness unless we also expand our moral awareness of right and wrong, good and evil. Later perhaps there will be ecstatic harmonies beyond the description of words in which the good and the evil of the world will be revealed as, mysteriously, the two hands of God. But only the soul that has honestly cast out violence, greed, and deception may begin the ascent to that lofty vision.[2]

Roszak, with his customary perceptiveness, continues:

Surely too many Western practitioners of yoga are playing trivial games with the psychic and physiological spin-off of the divine science. They learn to clear their sinuses, to mitigate their migraine, to flirt with the joys of the kundalini. Perhaps, besides achieving an enviable muscle tone, they even happen upon occasional intimations of samadhi. But all these achievements become barbarous trifles if we forget that yoga, like all spiritual culture, is a life discipline and a moral wisdom.[3]

The *Yoga-Sutra* of Patanjali mentions five moral precepts, which make up the category of *yama* ("discipline"), also called the "great vow" (*maha-vrata*). These five precepts, constituting the first "limb" of the eightfold yogic path delineated by Patanjali, are the following:

1. *Ahimsa*, or nonharming, which is nonmaliciousness in the broadest sense possible, extending to actions, thoughts, and speech. This is the most important rule of the moral code. The *yogin* who is thoroughly grounded in this virtue is surrounded by a peaceful aura that calms even wild beasts.

2. *Satya*, or truthfulness, about which the *Mahanirvana-Tantra* (IV.76) says that in its absence neither *mantra* recitation nor any other austerities can bear fruit. The Yoga practitioner who has mas-

tered this virtue is said to have the power of truth, so that all his or
her words come true.

3. *Asteya*, or nonstealing, which is defined in the *Yoga-Bhashya*
(II.30) as the unauthorized appropriation of another person's belongings. Mastery of this virtue is thought to bring to the *yogin* all
kinds of riches, both material and spiritual.

4. *Brahmacarya*, or chastity, which is explained in the *Yoga-
Bhashya* (II.30) as the control over the sexual organ. When the Yoga
practitioner is grounded in a chaste life, he or she gains great vitality
(*virya*), which facilitates concentration and spiritual life in general.

5. *Aparigraha*, or greedlessness, which Vyasa in his *Yoga-Bhashya*
(II.30) explains as the nonaquisition of things because one sees the
disadvantage in acquiring and keeping as well as losing or being
attached to them. Through perfection in greedlessness, adepts gain
insight into the reason for their own and others' births. The typical
Yoga adept lives very simply and frugally.

As Patanjali states in the *Yoga-Sutra* (II.31), these five virtues
must be cultivated irrespective of place, time, circumstance, or one's
social status. As a consequence, the powerful survival instinct is
rechanneled to serve a higher purpose. Practice of the five *yamas*
harmonizes the aspirant's social relationships and frees up a considerable amount of energy, which can then be invested in meditation
and the other advanced practices. Yoga practitioners do not choose
a moral way of life merely for their own convenience. Rather they
view their moral life as an obligation to the larger good by respecting
a cosmic pattern of harmony in which all beings can flourish and
find their true destiny.

The Five Practices of Self-Restraint

The second limb of the yogic path according to Patanjali is known
as *niyama* or "restraint." It stems from the same verbal root *yam*
("to restrain") from which *yama* is also derived. The prefix *ni-* is an
intensifier. This category consists of the following five practices:

1. *Shauca*, or purity, which refers not only to physical cleanliness but also to purity of the mind and speech. Yoga can be viewed as a protracted process of purification, which eliminates the dross of the ego-personality until only the radiant Self is evident.

2. *Samtosha*, or contentment, which the *Mahabharata* (XII.21.2) calls "the highest heaven." This is the practice of voluntary simplicity. The *Yoga-Bhashya* (II.32) explains it as "not to covet more than the means at hand." This, the *Yoga-Sutra* (II.42) states, makes for unexcelled joy.

3. *Tapas*, or austerity, which consists of all kinds of ascetic practices—from fasting and observing complete silence to standing stock-still for long periods of time. Such disciplines, apart from steeling the will, create an inner heat—also called *tapas*—which brings about a qualitative change in consciousness. According to the *Yoga-Sutra* (II.43), austerity causes all impurity of the body-mind to dwindle and leads to perfection of the body and the sense organs.

4. *Svadhyaya*, or study, which is generally understood as the study and recitation of the sacred texts, is said to lead to contact with one's chosen deity (*Yoga-Sutra* II.44). In his *Yoga-Varttika* commentary on Patanjali's aphorism, Vijnana Bhikshu explains that coming into contact means having the vision of a deity or a sage or other high master, who helps the *yogin* to accomplish his or her spiritual work.

5. *Ishvara-pranidhana*, or devotion to the Lord, which the *Yoga-Bhashya* (II.45) explains as dedicating all one's inner states to the Lord. In Patanjali's path, the Lord (*ishvara*) is considered to be a special kind of Self (*purusha*)—a Self that, unlike the Self of human beings, has never been subject to the illusion of being a limited ego-personality and therefore has also never accrued any karma. The fruit of devotion to the Lord is said to be the attainment of ecstasy (*samadhi*).

The five practices of *niyama* harness the energy generated from the consistent cultivation of the five moral disciplines. They increase the spiritual momentum in the *yogin's* life and prepare the ground for the other practices of the eightfold path.

The fifth practice, that of devotion to the Lord, deserves further commentary. Its presence in Patanjali's Raja-Yoga shows the supreme importance of the devotional element even in a path that centers on spiritual growth through wisdom. Some scholars have argued that the practice of devotion to the Lord was not originally part of Raja-Yoga, but this opinion is ill founded. It overlooks the fact that grace (*prasada*) has from the beginning been an inalienable aspect of the Yoga tradition. Even those schools that emphasize self-effort over grace do not completely deny that a great deal of help is extended to aspirants from the invisible dimension—whether through the agency of disembodied teachers, deities, or the Divine itself.

For Western practitioners of Yoga, perhaps the lesson in all this is to recognize that we are not isolated islands but part of a larger whole and that this whole is essentially benevolent. Those who make every effort on the path are inevitably supported by the higher powers. As Sri Aurobindo, the founding sage of Integral Yoga, put it:

> The Divine Grace is there ready to act at every moment, but
> it manifests as one grows out of the Law of Ignorance into
> the Law of Light.[4]

The Alchemy of Personal Transmutation

"A Yogi or a Jnani," wrote Swami Sivananda, "does not allow even a very small amount of energy in him to be wasted in useless directions."[5] Long before physicists discovered that matter is energy vibrating at a certain rate, the *yogins* of India had treated the human body-mind as a playful manifestation of the ultimate power (*shakti*), the dynamic aspect of Reality. They realized that to discover the true Self, one had to harness attention because the energy of the body-mind follows attention. A crude example of this process is the measurable increase of blood flow to our fingers and toes that occurs when we concentrate on them.

The *yogins* are very careful about where they place their attention, for the mind creates patterns of energy, causing habits of thought and behavior that can be detrimental to the pursuit of genuine happiness. Their goal is to always contemplate the Divine, or Self, until the mechanism of attention is freed from the mechanics of the body-mind and firmly anchored in the Self. Then a truly spontaneous life becomes possible—a life lived in the freedom of Self-realization.

The goal of conventional alchemy is to produce gold out of base metal. However, the goal of spiritual or esoteric alchemy has always been to generate a new state of being. The much-sought-after philosopher's stone was never a physical object but an inner realization—the realization of wisdom, gnosis, or *vidya*. Yoga is such a path of spiritual alchemy, consisting in the personal transmutation of the Yoga practitioner from a base, corrupted personality into the luminous, nonlocal Self beyond space and time.

5

Purification and Postures for Relaxation, Meditation, and Health

One should practice Yoga for the purification of the self.
—BHAGAVAD-GITA VI.12

The Body as a Temple of the Divine

The more ascetic schools of Yoga regard the body as a putrid heap of bones, sinews, and flesh. Yet all yogic authorities have acknowledged that embodied existence is precious, because it affords us a range of experiences that may trigger the impulse to seek enlightenment or liberation. Even the deities—corresponding to angelic beings in the Judeo-Christian tradition—are said to be at a disadvantage in this respect. Celestial life is too evenly delightful to be able to catapult the deities into the unconditional dimension of Reality, which alone stands for authentic freedom and lasting happiness. They may first have to take birth in a lower realm, including the physical world, to become liberated from the cycle of conditional existence (*samsara*).

Human life, then, is considered extremely precious in Yoga. In Tantrism and its offshoot Hatha-Yoga, the less-than-perfect body is even looked upon as a temple of the Divine (*deva-alaya*). The *Shiva-Samhita,* a seventeenth-century Hatha-Yoga text, contains the following verses:

46

This body (*gatra*), formed out of the five elements by the Creator, and known as the brahmic egg, is created for the experience of pleasure and pain. (I.95)

The conscious [Self] abiding in all beings experiences [pleasure and pain] by connecting with the unconscious [matter of the physical body]. Bound by its own karma, that which is known as the psyche (*jiva*) becomes multiple out of unconsciousness.

Karma is generated again and again in the so-called brahmic egg for experiences, and the psyche is dissolved when experience ends together with one's karma. (I.99–100)

When the body unconquered by karma is made an instrument [for attaining] *nirvana*,[1] then the bodily vehicle becomes worthwhile, not otherwise. (II.52)

The South Indian *yogin*-saint Tirumular included in his celebrated *Tirumandiram*, written in melodious Tamil, these two verses (here only paraphrased):

When the body perishes, the life force (*prana*) departs and the Light of Truth cannot be attained. I learned the art of preserving my body and thus also the life force in it.

Once I despised the body. But then I saw the Divine within it and realized the body is the Lord's temple. Thus I began to preserve it with great care. (verses 724–725)

The singular Self (*atman*), when it becomes karmically associated with a limited body and the finite universe, experiences itself as manifold psyches, each thinking it is an island unto itself. This delusion in turn generates the conditions for pleasurable and painful experiences, all of which are binding because they merely reinforce that initial delusion of mistaken identity. Only when all karma and limited experience is transcended does the individual psyche remember its true nature, as the singular Self manifesting in all beings and things.

The transition from ignorance to liberating wisdom, from the round of pleasure and pain to luminous happiness, is one of the simplest and yet most mysterious processes of existence. The *Shiva-Samhita* and many other scriptures, particularly of a Tantric nature, recommend an artful device to foster this process: to consciously remember oneself as the Self, as the Divine. Connected with this cognitive trick is the practical idea of viewing the human body as a replica of the cosmos at large. Thus the opening verses of the second chapter of the *Shiva-Samhita* describe how the cosmic mountain, Mount Meru, and the surrounding seven islands with their lakes, rivers, hills, plains, and presiding deities and sages, as well as the stars and planets, are all to be found within the human body. Hence the body is called the cosmic or brahmic egg (*brahma-anda*), from which all pleasant and unpleasant experiences hatch. Yoga is the means of cracking the egg and thus escaping its karmic inevitabilities.

Cracking the egg, however, is a subtle process. It cannot be accomplished by merely killing off the body, which would be a karmic act leading to the creation of another body and very likely more difficult experiences. Only wisdom can end this vicious circle of karmic self-reproduction.

The *yogins* look at the larger picture, viewing their actions in the light of not only this present birth but all future embodiments as well. In fact, they endeavor to lop off the karmic tree at its roots to terminate the cycle of countless rebirths. They strive to be free once and for all.

The idea of reincarnation, which goes hand in hand with the belief in karma, is fundamental to traditional Yoga and the other liberation teachings of India. Some newcomers to Yoga have difficulty believing that their present life is merely one link in a long chain of embodiments. They might be helped in their consideration of this metaphysical notion by reading Arthur and Joyce Berger's book *Reincarnation: Fact or Fable?* and Joseph Head and S. L. Cranston's compilation *Reincarnation: An East-West Anthology*.² But even those who do not see the intrinsic reasonableness of this ancient belief, or prefer to suspend judgment about it, can still practice Yoga successfuly so long as they understand the workings of the law of cause and effect in the moral realm: We reap as we sow.

The Groundwork of Bodily Purification

The yogic path can be viewed as a lengthy process of physical and mental purification, or catharsis. According to the *Yoga-Sutra* (III.55), the Self shines forth when the highest aspect of the mind, the *sattva*, approximates the Self in purity. Hence the *yogin* makes every effort to polish the mirror of the mind so as to reflect the light of the Self without distortion. The Yoga authorities long ago recognized the intimate relationship between the body and the mind. Therefore Hatha-Yoga entails a fairly complex program of physical cleansing (*shodhana*) that is meant to support the *yogin's* inner work of self-purification through meditation and ecstatic absorption.

The *Gheranda-Samhita* describes the following "six acts" (*shat-karma*) of bodily purification:

1. *Dhauti* ("cleansing") consists of four techniques: (a) inner cleansing (*antar-dhauti*), (b) dental cleansing (*danta-dhauti*), (c) "heart cleansing" (*hrid-dhauti*), and (d) "base purification" (*mula-shodhana*). Inner cleansing comprises four exercises: swallowing the breath and expelling it through the anus; filling the stomach with water; stimulating the "fire" in the abdomen through repeatedly pushing the navel back against the spine; and washing the prolapsed intestines (a rather dangerous practice). Dental cleansing covers cleaning the teeth, tongue, ears, and frontal sinuses. Heart cleansing consists in cleansing the throat by means of a plantain stalk, turmeric, a cane, or a piece of cloth, or by self-induced vomiting. Here the word *hrid* ("heart") stands for "chest." Base purifica-

tion is the manual cleansing of the anus with water or some other natural substance.

2. *Vasti* ("bladder") is the contraction and dilation of the sphincter muscle and is often performed while standing in water.

3. *Neti* (untranslatable) refers to the practice of inserting a thin thread about nine inches in length into the nose and passing it through the mouth. This fairly simple practice is said to remove phlegm and open up the "third eye"—that is, activate the *ajna-cakra* in the middle of the forehead, thus giving rise to clairvoyant abilities.

4. *Lauli* ("to-and-fro movement"), also called *nauli*, consists in rolling the abdominal muscles sideways to massage the stomach, intestines, and other inner organs.

5. *Trataka* (untranslatable) is the steady, relaxed gazing at a small object, such as the flame of a candle, until tears begin to flow. This is thought to improve one's eyesight and induce clairvoyance.

6. *Kapala-bhati* ("skull luster") comprises the following three practices, which are said to reduce phlegm: (a) The "left process" (*vama-krama*) consists in breathing through the left nostril and expelling the air through the right and vice versa; (b) the "inverted process" (*vyut-krama*) consists in drawing water up through the nostrils and expelling it through the mouth (which is a form of *neti*); and (c) the "*shit* process" (*shit-krama*) consists in sucking water up through the mouth and expelling it through the nose, which makes the sound *shit*, after which the practice is named.

Other manuals describe these purificatory techniques differently and add further exercises to the repertoire of preparatory practices. Like almost all Yoga practices, they are best learned from a competent teacher. They rid the body of impurities and prepare it for the cultivation of the postures (*asana*) and other practices, especially meditation. A toxic body interferes with inner harmony and balance. Particularly in Hatha-Yoga, the "forceful" Yoga, physical impurities can cause unpleasant symptoms in the nervous system when the serpent power, or *kundalini-shakti*, is activated.

Relaxation Is Liberating

Relaxation is the alpha and omega of Yoga. How so? According to the yogic worldview, ordinary life, revolving around the accumulation of pleasurable and painful experiences, is a result of the contraction of consciousness. In its pure state, as the transcendental Self, consciousness is completely unrestricted and free. However, through wrongful identification with a particular body-mind, the spacious consciousness of the Self seemingly contracts to create the limited awareness of the psyche (*jiva*). In truth, the Self never contracts at all. The illusion of contraction is the problem. Yoga therefore seeks to undermine this illusion by which all unenlightened beings bind themselves. It endeavors to systematically remove all those binds that help maintain the illusion. This endeavor can be viewed as an extensive process of disentanglement, or purification, or relaxation.

In this broader sense, relaxation denotes letting go of the tension that creates the illusion of the ego's individuality and separateness. Thus relaxation is not merely relaxation of the body but also of the mind—our opinions, concerns, hopes, and attitudes. It is the master key to all levels of the yogic enterprise. But for most people, bodily relaxation is an excellent starting point for this more comprehensive process of letting go.

Interestingly, in the *Yoga-Sutra* Patanjali describes relaxation as the very essence of the yogic postures (*asana*). He uses the term *shaithilya*, which means "loosening." He explains:

> Posture [should be] steady and comfortable.
> [It should be accompanied] by the loosening of tension (*prayatna*) and by coinciding with the infinite [space of consciousness]. (II.45–46)

When posture is cultivated properly, it yields the peculiar sensation that the body—or rather our felt image of it—is loosening up or widening out. Hence Patanjali speaks of one's consciously coinciding with the infinite (*ananta*), by which he probably means the infinite space of consciousness opening up before us as we get closer to our authentic identity, the Self. Thus posture is much more than gymnastics or acrobatics. It is the art of relaxation to the point of meditation and beyond. When a posture is practiced successfully, the practitioner inevitably has the sensation of extending beyond the skin, of being a vibrant energy field that imperceptibly merges with the environment.

As a result of this, the practitioner becomes, as Patanjali puts it in his *Yoga-Sutra* (II.48), unassailable by the play of dualities such as heat and cold, humidity and aridity, or pleasure and pain. In other words, the *yogin* acquires the first degree of sensory inhibition (*pratyahara*), which also is a separate yogic practice on the eightfold path.

For Patanjali, who probably lived in the second century CE (though some scholars place him before the common era), posture still meant meditation posture. With the appearance of Hatha-Yoga, posture was given the additional function of restoring or maintaining bodily health. The thought behind the new approach was this: If the body is a temple of the Divine and a unique opportunity for achieving liberation, we must do our best to keep it clean and in optimal condition. Hatha-Yoga includes numerous techniques of bodily cleansing and energetic purification. They all are designed to promote relaxation in the broader sense introduced here and ultimately to lead to enlightenment.

The Sanskrit word *asana* means literally "seat" and on occasion is used to designate just that. But in yogic contexts, the term is primarily employed to refer to the typical Yoga postures. That yogic posture stands for more than a mere bodily pose is indicated by the fact that the texts also use the synonym *pitha*. Ordinarily, this word is reserved for a shrine or sacred place. This suggests that a yogic posture is a sacred act, which transforms the body into a shrine for inner worship. Mircea Eliade grasped this symbolic aspect of *asana* perhaps better than most. He wrote that:

asana is the first concrete step taken for the purpose of abol-
ishing the modalities of human existence. What is certain is
that the motionless, hieratic position of the body imitates
some other condition than the human; the yogin in the state
of *asana* can be homologized with a plant or a sacred statue.[3]

In other words, *asana* is the initial effort to construct a divine
body, or to honor the fact that the body is a temple of the Divine.
Divorced from this spiritual orientation, the yogic postures cannot,
as Sri Aurobindo observed, cure the body "of that restlessness which
is a sign of its inability to contain without working them off in action
and movement the vital forces poured into it from the universal Life-
Ocean."[4]

Postures for Meditation

Because meditation requires that we sit still for a long span of
time, it is important that we find a comfortable position that supports our inner work. Perhaps the most comfortable position is the
corpse posture (*shava-asana*), which often concludes a postural se-
quence. Also known as the dead pose, this *asana* is excellent for
relaxation. Yet it is not particularly suitable for meditation, because
we associate this pose with sleep, and, unless we have achieved a
certain degree of expertise in meditation, the corpse posture invites
sleep rather than mental lucidity.

Most Hatha-Yoga manuals favor the following two *asanas* for meditation:

1. *Siddha-asana* ("adept's posture") is executed by pressing the
left heel against the perineum and placing the other foot above the
genitals. When the right heel is pressed against the perineum, with
the other foot placed above the genitals, this posture is also called
vajra-asana in some texts. The *Hatha-Yoga-Pradipika* asks, "When
siddha-asana is mastered, of what use are the various other pos-

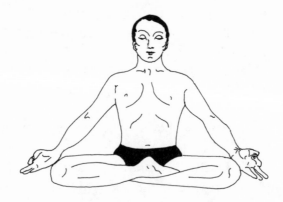

Siddha-asana ("adept's posture")

tures?" (I.41) This shows the high esteem in which the adept's posture is held in Hatha-Yoga circles.

2. *Padma-asana* ("lotus posture") is performed by placing the
right foot on the left thigh and the left foot on the right thigh. The
classical manuals also instruct the practitioner to cross the arms behind the back and grasp the left toe with the left hand and the right
toe with the right hand. This variation is also called the bound lotus
posture (*baddha-padma-asana*). "After the initial knee pains have
been overcome," remarks B. K. S. Iyengar, "padmasana is one of
the most relaxing poses."[5] Apart from being an excellent posture for
prolonged meditation, the lotus posture also is said to remove a variety of diseases. It is most frequently seen in depictions of the Buddha, who was not only an enlightened being but also a great master
of meditation.

A third posture, favored by many Western students, is the *sukha-
asana* ("pleasant posture"), which is widely known as the tailor's
seat. This posture is easy on the knees but not very stable for longer
periods of meditation.

It should be noted here that the Sanskrit texts do not always use
the same name for the same exercise, which has led to a certain
amount of confusion among students. Thus in some manuals the

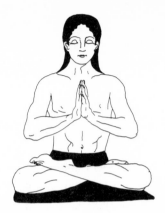

Padma-asana ("lotus posture")

sukha-asana goes by the name *svastika-asana*, while the *siddha-asana* is also called *vajra-asana*, *mukta-asana* ("liberated posture"), or *gupta-asana* ("concealed posture"). Moreover, the same posture may be performed with subtle but significant differences in the various schools. In light of this, it is obviously important to pay close attention to the descriptions provided in textbooks or by one's teacher.

Classical Postures for Health Maintenance and Therapy

The Hatha-Yoga scriptures state that there are 840,000 natural bodily positions. Of these, eight-four postures constitute the classical set of *asanas*, described in later manuals. This elaborate set was arrived at gradually in the course of many centuries of intensive practical experimentation.

In the *Gheranda-Samhita*, of the late seventeenth century, only thirty-two postures are described. By contrast, some modern works list and depict over two hundred *asanas*. Western Yoga teachers have made their greatest contribution to the yogic tradition by adapting the classical postures to the special needs and abilities of their students. In particular, they have done much to refine the preparatory stages leading up to the classical postures. However, because of its emphasis on postures and its deemphasis of the traditional spiritual value system, Western Hatha-Yoga often lacks the depth of its Indian counterpart. Yet even India has produced its share of practitioners who mistake Yoga for fitness training or acrobatics. This prompted Sri Aurobindo to speak of the "exorbitant price" paid by Hatha-Yoga practitioners, who spend endless years in full-time training often "to very little purpose."[6]

The following is a selection of some of the better-known *asanas:*

1. *Vriksha-asana* ("tree posture") is done by balancing on one leg in the standing position. The foot of the other leg is propped against the standing leg near the knee or higher. The arms are extended upward, with the palms together. This posture has numerous variants.

2. *Trikona-asana* ("triangle posture") is a sideways bend of the upper body while standing with legs wide apart and with arms extended at a right angle from the trunk.

3. *Pada-hasta-asana* ("hands-to-feet posture") is a forward bend

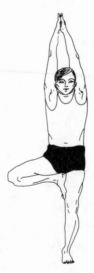

Vriksha-asana ("tree posture")

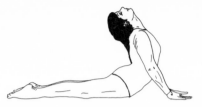

Bhujanga-asana ("serpent posture")

from the standing position, with the hands grasping the feet and the face (if easily possible) touching the legs.

4. *Vajra-asana* ("adamantine posture" or "thunderbolt posture") is done by sitting down between the feet, which rest to either side of the buttocks.

5. *Go-mukha-asana* ("cow-face posture") is performed in the adamantine posture, with alternately one hand reaching down over the shoulder and grasping the hand of the other arm, which is reaching upward between the shoulder blades.

6. *Pashcima-uttana-asana* ("back-stretching posture") is done while being seated with legs outstretched next to each other and bending forward. The hands grasp the feet, and the face rests on the knees.

7. *Bhujanga-asana* ("serpent posture," popularly "cobra pose") is done by lying on the stomach and pushing the upper body upward with the arms.

8. *Sarva-anga-asana* ("all-limb posture," better known as the shoulderstand) is executed by extending the legs upward while supporting the back with the hands.

9. *Hala-asana* ("plow posture") can be performed from the position of the shoulderstand by bringing the legs up over the head until the feet touch the ground, while supporting the pelvis with the arms.

10. *Shirsha-asana* ("head posture," better known as the headstand) is a powerful inversion exercise that should be assumed with the utmost caution. It is done by placing the top of the head on the

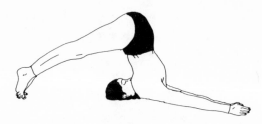

Hala-asana ("plow posture")

ground, with the neck supported by the arms, and slowly raising the legs upward. This practice should not be imitated from a book or video.

Most of the postures for health maintenance or restoration are executed deliberately and slowly, with great inner awareness and collectedness. The Indian Yoga researcher M. V. Bhole characterized the yogic postures as "molds," "casts," or "patterns," because "they are to be maintained for a certain length of time in a passive manner with an emphasis to achieve relaxation of those muscles involved in assuming the posture itself."[7] Thus the postures are psychophysical templates promoting symmetry, balance, and harmony, as well as inner peace.

The most important aspect of *asana* practice, to which Western students do not always pay sufficient attention, is the proper regulation of the breath. Some postures call for deep, even breathing, or the holding of the breath, or even rapid shallow breathing. Clearly, the postures and their correct sequencing should be learned from a qualified teacher.

Bandhas and Mudras: Sealing the Body's Energy

A special type of posture is exemplified by the various *bandhas* and *mudras*. The Sanskrit word *bandha* means "bond," or, in the present context, "lock." Hatha-Yoga recognizes the following three principal locks by which the life force (*prana*) is forcibly retained in the body:

1. *Mula-bandha* ("root lock") is the contraction of the sphincter muscle, also known as *ashvini-mudra* ("horse seal"). Some manuals describe the root lock differently.

2. *Uddiyana-bandha* ("upward lock") is generally executed by exhaling and pulling the stomach up until there is a hollow below the rib cage. This technique is said to force the vital energy upward like a great bird.

3. *Jalandhara-bandha* ("Jalandhara's lock") is also called *kantha-samkocana* or "throat contraction." It is done by pushing the chin down against the collar bone. This technique stops the downward flow of the ambrosial liquid (possibly a reference to a hormonal secretion) generated at the palate. But it also prevents the life energy (and the breath) from leaving the body through the mouth or the nose.

These three locks are usually applied together but can be practiced separately as well.

The Sanskrit term *mudra* means "seal." In Hatha-Yoga, a *mudra* is a specific type of posture involving a more deliberate manipulation of the life force than in the case of the other *asanas*. The *Gheranda-Samhita* speaks of twenty-five seals, including the three locks, the shoulderstand (here called *viparita-karani-mudra*), and five meditation exercises involving visualization of the five material elements—earth, water, fire, air, and ether/space.

The eight most important seals found in the Hatha-Yoga literature are the following:

1. *Khecari-mudra* ("space-walking seal"),[8] a most important technique in Hatha-Yoga, is performed by turning the tongue back and inserting it into the cavity leading to the nose. This is possible only when the tendon (frenum) underneath the tongue has been cut. This *mudra* is said to still hunger, quench thirst, cure all kinds of

diseases, and even conquer death. This practice is also known as *nabho-mudra* ("space seal").

2. *Shakti-calani-mudra* ("power-stirring seal") is done while seated in the *siddha-asana* and involves contracting the sphincter muscle and focusing the life force into the central channel (*sushumna-nadi*) at the lowest psychoenergetic center, the seat of the serpent power.

3. *Shambhavi-mudra* ("Shambhu's seal") is not so much a physical exercise as a meditation technique. It involves an unfocused gazing with wide open eyes while contemplating the infinite. Shambhu is another name for Shiva, who is regarded as the original revealer of the secrets of Tantrism.

4. *Vajroli-mudra* (untranslatable), according to the *Hatha-Yoga-Pradipika* (III.85ff.), is done by sucking the released semen back into the urethra. Female practitioners also can learn this technique, which was invented so as not to waste the valuable hormonal and chemical properties of semen. Other texts give this exercise a nonsexual connotation.

5. *Sahajoli-mudra* (untranslatable), again according to the *Hatha-Yoga-Pradipika* (III.93), consists in rubbing ejaculated semen into the skin.

6. *Amaroli-mudra* (untranslatable) is what in the West is called "urine therapy," consisting in drinking the midflow of the urine, thought to have healing properties. The term *amaroli* contains the word *amara* ("immortal"), meaning the nectar of immortality, which is the esoteric name for the urine.

7. *Yoni-mudra* ("womb seal") is executed while seated in the *siddha-asana*, with eyes, ears, and nostrils closed with the ten fingers. It consists essentially in forcing the life energy (*prana*) through the six psychoenergetic centers (*cakra*) of the body by means of breath control, *mantra* recitation, and visualization. Some authorities equate the womb seal with the six-openings seal, while others equate it with

the horse seal (*ashvini-mudra*), which is the contraction of the sphincter muscle.

8. *Shan-mukhi-mudra* ("six-openings seal") is done by placing the thumbs on the two ears, the index and middle fingers on the two eyes, and the ring and little fingers on the two nostrils. Sometimes practitioners are instructed to place the little fingers near or on the upper lip.

It is evident from these descriptions that these yogic seals mark an important transition phase from the more physically oriented postures to the techniques of breath control (*prana* manipulation) and meditation. Little wonder that Svatmarama Yogindra, the author of the *Hatha-Yoga-Pradipika*, felt called to make this claim for the yogic seals:

> One who gives traditional instruction about the seals, he indeed is a blessed (*shri*) teacher. He indeed is a master (*svamin*), the Lord in person.
>
> He who concentrates on the practice of the seals, following the teaching of that [blessed teacher], quickly obtains the [paranormal] qualities such as miniaturization (*animan*) [but more important he] defeats time [that is, conquers death]. (III.129–130)

The adept (*siddha*) is traditionally portrayed as someone who has attained spiritual perfection (*siddhi*) and who also is a thaumaturgist possessing all the great paranormal powers (*siddhi*). The capacity of "miniaturization" spoken of in the above passage is an adept's ability to make himself or herself as small as an atom. This and other similar abilities must be understood as applying to the subtle body rather than the physical body, which is also how some Sanskrit texts understand it.

6

Yogic Diet

Yoga is not for him who overeats and also not for him who does not eat.

—BHAGAVAD-GITA VI.16

Food for Health and Wholeness

Like any other system of integral well-being, Yoga includes more or less specific dietary rules. Most of Yoga's dietary wisdom is transmitted by word of mouth. However, some general rules, as well as some specific instructions, can be found in various Sanskrit scriptures. The reason *yogins* have since ancient times paid close attention to diet is expressed in a nutshell in the archaic *Chandogya-Upanishad* (VI.5.4), which speaks of the mind as being "composed of food" (*anna-maya*). According to this teaching, the coarsest part of food is eliminated through the digestive tract, its less coarse part is turned into flesh (that is, sustains the body), while its subtle aspect becomes mind (that is, feeds our nervous system and the brain processes). The mind sustained by food is known as the lower mind, called *manas*. Food does not go into the making of the higher mind, or *buddhi*, which is the seat or source of wisdom.

In the same Upanishadic passage, the coarsest part of water is transmuted into urine, its less coarse part becomes blood, while its subtle aspect goes to form the breath.

In later times, this whole notion came to be expressed in the popular Indian maxim, "As one's food, so is one's mind" (*yatha annam tatha manah*). This resonates with the well-known declaration of the nineteenth-century German philosopher Ludwig Feuerbach, who said that "man is what he eats." In India, of course, this is held to be true only of the body-mind, whereas the spirit or Self remains completely unaffected by our dietary habits.

Yet, how we relate to the Self, our innermost nature, is to some extent affected by what (and also how) we eat. In other words, the biochemical conditions of the body are significant in the process of yogic self-transformation, and eating is an important influence on our body chemistry and state of mind. An extreme example of the close link between our mental state and the substances we introduce into our body is the consumption of alcohol and other such drugs. They chemically alter our blood and our mental functioning. The substances we call food have a similar, if less dramatic, effect. Most of us have experienced sugar highs and subsequent lows. Likewise, most of us know the physical and emotional feeling of being weighed down from overeating. Some of us have experienced the clarity and alertness that come with fasting for several days.

Nutrition is increasingly recognized as a significant factor in health maintenance. The practitioners of Ayur-Veda, the native Indian system of health care, realized this long ago. Their wisdom spilled over into Yoga, and Yoga in turn influenced Ayur-Veda. The primary purpose of diet in Yoga, however, is not merely to maintain or restore physical health but to keep the inner environment, the mind, free from pollution. In the *Bhagavad-Gita*, composed twenty-five hundred years ago, we find the following threefold classification of food:

> Foods that promote life, the lucidity-factor (*sattva*), strength, health, happiness, and satisfaction and are savory,

oil-rich, firm, and hearty—these are agreeable to the *sattva*-natured [person].

Foods that are pungent, sour, salty, hot, sharp, harsh, and burning—these are coveted by the *rajas*-natured [person]. They cause pain, grief, and disease.

And [food] that is spoiled, tasteless, putrid, stale, left over, and unclean—this is food agreeable to the *tamas*-natured [person]. (XVII.8–10)

This threefold division of food according to the three qualities of Nature—*sattva* (lucidity), *rajas* (dynamism), and *tamas* (inertia)—also is adhered to by later Hindu authorities. Occasionally, the scriptures are more specific, mentioning particular plants and other food items suitable or unsuitable for the *yogin*. For example, in the *Hatha-Yoga-Pradipika* (I.59ff.), green vegetables, sour gruel, oil, sesamum, mustard, alcohol, fish, meat, oil cake, asafetida, and garlic are listed as unsalutary foods. However, wheat, rice, barley, certain cucumbers, potherbs, green gram (mung beans), butter, brown sugar, honey, milk, and ghee (clarified butter) are recommended.

Western Yoga students may not find such food lists helpful, and many prefer to follow modern holistic nutrition. Who, however, could find fault with the yogic recommendation to practice moderate eating (*mita-ahara*), which is frequently counted among the practices of moral restraint (*yama*)? Overeating is a form of stealing, and it is probably the single most detrimental factor in our Western dietary habits. The yogic practice of periodic fasting (*upavasa*) is also an excellent way of maintaining and restoring one's health, as more and more physicians have become willing to admit.

The Yoga scriptures especially emphasize the need for moderate eating and warn that overeating causes all kinds of diseases and prevents ultimate success in Yoga. At the same time, the Tantric scriptures observe that in the present dark age, people tend to turn to food for meaning and consolation. We must therefore be doubly watchful of our culinary habits.

Yet, certain dietary rules stated in the Yoga scriptures would seem to make sense only in a strictly traditional setting and in the specific context of India's flora. While the broad guidelines given in the Yoga texts are valid, it is also true that one's diet should be tailored to one's individual requirements. Experimentation with one's nutrition and learning to listen to the wisdom of the body are therefore advisable. Physician and Yoga practitioner Rudolph Ballentine, who is a student of Swami Rama, has compiled a comprehensive guide entitled *Diet and Nutrition: A Holistic Approach.*[1] This and similar works offer the kind of detailed, sensible advice that can be most helpful to conscientious practitioners of Yoga living in the West.

Vegetarianism

Yogins, like most Hindus, are typically lacto-vegetarians, balancing their intake of fruit, vegetables, grains, and nuts with milk and milk products. Only the initiates of left-hand Tantrism consume meat as a sacrament during their secret gatherings. The *yogins* of Buddhism—with the exception of Tibetan Buddhism—likewise abstain from eating meat. Some are vegans—omitting all animal products from their diet—and a few are fruitarians. They all have in common a minimalist approach to eating.

The reason for vegetarianism in Hinduism and Buddhism is largely philosophical and ethical, but health is also a consideration. Hindus and Buddhists, as well as the adherents of Jainism, uphold the moral virtue of nonharming (*ahimsa*) and consequently abhor killing for food. They believe that slaughtering an animal has karmic consequences for oneself, and the more spiritually aware a person is, the more serious those consequences will be. Also, eating meat is thought to transfer something of the animal's coarse qualities to the eater. In contemporary Yoga circles, this is usually expressed in terms of the low vibration of animal flesh.

Mahatma Gandhi, who was an exemplary *karma-yogin*, believed he owed his physical fitness not only to his detachment but also to his strict adherence to regular habits in eating, drinking, and sleeping. Well known for his dietary experiments, he admitted that there is no fixed dietary rule applying to all constitutions with equal force. "The popular saying," he wrote, "that one man's food may be another's poison is based on vast experience which finds daily verification."[2] Nevertheless, Gandhi also observed: "Diet is a powerful factor not to be neglected. . . . Vegetarianism is one of the priceless gifts of Hinduism."[3] Gandhi made it very clear that, unless one feels naturally drawn to a vegetarian diet, one must cultivate a strong moral conviction. As he put it:

> For remaining staunch to vegetarianism a man requires a moral basis. . . . Because it is for the building of the spirit and not of the body. Man is more than meat. It is the spirit in man for which we are concerned. Therefore, vegetarians should have that moral basis—that a man was not born a carnivorous animal, but born to live on the fruits and herbs that the earth grows.[4]

Today the medical establishment is beginning to recognize the health advantages of a diet restricted in meat and other animal products. A growing number of physicians are even slowly questioning the widely proclaimed benefits of milk and milk products, as many people seem to be allergic to them. Only personal experimentation can tell the Yoga practitioner which foods are suitable for his or her constitution and promote the *sattva* element, leading to increased bodily, emotional, and mental well-being.

The Yoga of Eating

As important as the food we eat, if not more so, is the manner in which we eat. Any activity in which we engage semiconsciously, without attentiveness, merely perpetuates our unconscious patterns and thus our condition of unenlightenment and suffering. This holds true also of the way in which we consume our food. We may eat a delicious vegetarian meal—prepared from the healthiest, most nutritious ingredients, and full of Nature's goodness. Yet, if we gulp down our food unthinkingly or indifferently, perhaps while watching television, we miss the opportunity for yogic practice that every meal affords us. For the Yoga of eating demands that we consciously participate in the process of feeding our body, so that we simultaneously feed our inner being. This idea has been poignantly expressed by the contemporary adept Omraam Mikhael Aivanhov, a master of Surya-Yoga (Solar Yoga):

> To receive the most subtle particles in the food, you must be fully conscious, wide awake, full of love. If the entire system is ready to receive food in that perfect way, then the food is moved to pour out its hidden riches . . . when food opens itself, it gives you all that it has in the way of pure, divine energies.[5]

Aivanhov further stated:

> I will tell you what an Initiate does. First of all, knowing that he must prepare the best possible conditions in order to benefit from the elements Nature has prepared, he begins by recollecting himself, remaining silent and devoting his thoughts to his Creator. . . . He knows also that the first mouthful is most important (the most important moment of any action is the first step) for it signals the release of forces which once released do not stop but continue to the end: if you begin in a state of harmony, whatever you do will be harmonious to the end.
>
> And then he eats slowly and chews the food thoroughly, not only for the sake of his digestion, but because the mouth is a spiritual laboratory which absorbs the subtle etheric energies before sending the grosser particles on down to the stomach.[6]

In addition to this inner concentration, Aivanhov explained, initiates also cultivate feelings of gratitude, which "transform gross matter into light and joy."[7] Traditionally, such gratitude is expressed by offering a portion of one's food to the Divine. Thus the *Bhagavad-Gita* (III.13) declares that those who cook merely for themselves—that is, who do not understand the obligation of gratitude and offerings—are but thieves.

For Aivanhov, nutrition is a form of conception—the birth of thoughts or moods that will either harmonize our being or throw it into chaos and distress. Although Aivanhov was a Bulgarian gnostic, his teaching on this point is in essential agreement with the Yoga tradition, with which he was familiar. What he taught explicitly is implicit in all yogic teachings, which recommend not only moderate eating (*mita-ahara*) but also disciplined eating (*yukta-ahara*). And discipline in the intake of nourishment means first and foremost bringing full awareness to this important aspect of life.

7

The Breath: Secret Bridge to Vitality and Bliss

Entering the Earth, I support all beings by [My] vitality (ojas).
—BHAGAVAD-GITA XV.13

The Multidimensional Body

To understand the practice of breath control, the fourth limb of the eightfold yogic path, we must first appreciate that the body is merely the outermost level or layer of the multidimensional structure that constitutes what we call the "human being." Likewise the breath is only the external aspect of the universal life force (*prana*), whose deepest root is Life or the ultimate Reality itself. According to an ancient model, the life force forms a particular field around the physical body, creating a bridge between the body and the mind. Thus yogic breath control is not simply manipulation of the intake of oxygen into our lungs but a technique for regulating the flow of life force and, in codependence, the mental processes.

In Yoga practice, breath control equals mental control. This formula is as fundamental as Einstein's equation $E = mc^2$, and as far-reaching in its practical implications. It is through the proper regulation of the life force that the *yogin* can not only influence the nervous system and bodily functioning in general but also gain access to the subtle dimensions of existence by transcending the brain-dependent activities of the mind.

According to a very old teaching, found in the *Taittiriya-Upanishad* (II.2–5), the embodied human being exists simultaneously on five levels, called "envelopes" (*kosha*). In ascending order, these are:

1. *Anna-maya-kosha* ("envelope consisting of food"), which is the material body (*deha*)
2. *Prana-maya-kosha* ("envelope consisting of life force"), which is the bioenergetic field surrounding the material body
3. *Mano-maya-kosha* ("envelope consisting of mind"), which is the "lower" mind (*manas*), serving as a processor for all sensory input
4. *Vijnana-maya-kosha* ("envelope consisting of intelligence"), which is the "higher" mind or *buddhi*, the seat of discriminative understanding and wisdom
5. *Ananda-maya-kosha* ("envelope consisting of bliss"), which is that energetic field through which the individual connects with the ultimate Reality, which is inherently blissful

According to Shankara, the greatest exponent of Advaita Vedanta, the *ananda-maya-kosha* is identical not with the ultimate Reality but with the final veil of ignorance that separates the psyche from the transcendental Self, or ultimate Reality.[1] The Self is our true nature, which transcends the five envelopes or casings. This teaching is born from the ancient sages' versatile experience of ecstatic states, and there is virtually nothing in our everyday life that could help us understand it. The bliss that floods the psyche in high states of ecstasy has no parallel. Even the thrill of orgasm, which some experience with great intensity, pales by comparison with the bliss (*ananda*) of coming near, never mind merging with, the Self. In some respects, the word "bliss" is even misleading when applied to the Self. Bliss is still an experience, whereas Self-realization is not an experience but a mind- and body-transcending event, namely the recovery of our true identity.

Riding the Breath to Bliss

Whatever we contemplate or place our attention on, that we become. This is a profound piece of wisdom, first expressed in the Upanishads, which is fundamental to the practice of Yoga and Vedanta. What it means is that attention is a decisive factor in how we experience the world we live in. Walking down Main Street, a visiting sports enthusiast will easily spot a gym among the many stores but fail to see an antiquarian bookstore that promptly catches the booklover's eye. A child is apt to spot a toy store long before the parents, and an adult male might not see the little boutique until the fashion-conscious woman accompanying him steers toward it. A criminal will notice which stores have burglar alarms and which do not. Our attention informs the choices or decisions we make, and they in turn shape our attention and the quality of our existence.

According to the Indian sages, the ordinary person focuses his or her attention on ephemeral things and therefore does not invest energy in what they consider the only worthwhile pursuit—the pursuit of lasting happiness through realization of the Self (*atman*). By contrast, they themselves have attention only for the Self and therefore would score extremely low on any scale measuring worldly ambition. But because of their single-minded focus on the Self, they in fact realize, or *become*, the Self. The ordinary person, however, continues to animate the ego-personality and thus remains subject to unhappiness and suffering.

Having understood the destiny-making power of attention, the *yogins* do their utmost to cultivate vigilance over the mind. In this endeavor they enlist the help of the breath. As Swami Vivekananda put it:

In this body of ours, the breath motion is the "silent thread";
by laying hold of and learning to control it we grasp the pack
thread of the nerve currents, and from these the stout twine
of our thoughts, and lastly the rope of prana, controlling
which we reach freedom.[2]

Vivekananda's imagery has its roots in the Sanskrit scriptures, as
is evident from the following verses from the *Goraksha-Paddhati*
(Footsteps of Goraksha):

Even as a hawk, tied to a rope, can be brought back again
[when it has] flown off—thus the [principle of] life, bound
to the *gunas*, is pulled about by the in-breath and the out-
breath. (I.40)

Even as a ball, struck with a club, flies up—thus the [prin-
ciple of] life (*jiva*), similarly struck by the in-breath (*prana*)
and the out-breath (*apana*), does not rest.

Under the influence of the in-breath and the out-breath,
the [principle of] life rushes up and down through the left
and the right path. Because of this moving-to-and-fro it cannot be seen. (I.38–39)

The word *guna* means "strand" and refers to the three qualities of
Nature, which weave the web of conditional existence: *tamas* (the
principle of inertia), *rajas* (the dynamic principle), and *sattva* (the
principle of luminosity). These three *gunas* are thought to bind the
psyche via the mechanism of the breath. Yet the breath is also the
secret key to liberation, or enlightenment, because by controlling it,
the inner world of psyche and mind can also be brought under control and thus the portal to the Self can be opened.

Writing shortly after World War II about the Kriya-Yoga taught to
him by Sri Yukteswar, Paramahansa Yogananda observed in his popular *Autobiography of a Yogi*:

By *Kriya*, the outgoing life force is not wasted and abused
in the senses, but constrained to reunite with subtler spinal

energies. By such reinforcement of life, the yogi's body and brain cells are electrified with the spiritual elixir. . . . Untying the cord of breath which binds the soul to the body, *Kriya* serves to prolong life and enlarge the consciousness of infinity. The yoga method overcomes the tug of war between the mind and the matter-bound senses, and frees the devotee to reinherit his eternal kingdom. He knows his real nature is bound neither by physical encasement nor by breath, symbol of the mortal enslavement to air, to nature's elemental compulsions.[3]

Yogananda's comments about breath control through Kriya-Yoga apply equally to other yogic approaches involving *pranayama*. As is clear from his explanations, this similarity in the theory and practice of breath control in the various schools of Yoga is due to the thoroughly empirical orientation espoused in all of them.

Swami Rama, a contemporary exponent of Yoga, reiterates the traditional view when he writes:

Breath is an external manifestation of the force of *prana*. Breath is the fly-wheel that regulates the entire machine of the body. Just as the control of the fly-wheel of an engine controls all other mechanisms in it, so the control of the external breath leads to control of the gross and subtle, physical and mental aspects of our life machine.[4]

Ordinarily our breathing is quite irregular, just as our mental activity consists for the most part of a discontinuous, haphazard flux of thoughts, rising and disappearing like flashes of lightning. Moreover, like our breath, our thoughts are seldom very deep. According to the yogic point of view, erratic and shallow breathing makes for erratic and shallow thinking. Interestingly, when we concentrate we often hold our breath. In Yoga, breath retention has been made into a fine art.

Pranayama as Life Extension

The term *pranayama* is composed of *prana* ("life," "life force") and *ayama* ("extension"), thus meaning the lengthening of breath, vital energy, and even life itself. Although some researchers have tried to demythologize the age-old notion of *prana* by reducing it to mere oxygen, when the ancient authorities speak of *prana* they always understand it to be air or breath plus Factor X—a kind of universal energy whose irradiant quality can be experienced by the sensitive Yoga practitioner.

The rolling waves or oscillations of the life force manifest themselves in the body in the breathing rhythm, which is a semiautomatic response. It is a vital function of the organism and is partly controlled by the autonomic nervous system. However, unlike the heartbeat or the peristalsis of the intestines, which are involuntary physiological processes, breathing can be consciously influenced to a considerable degree; it can be modified and even stopped completely for an appreciable span of time. In the late nineteenth century, a *yogin* going by the name of Haridas baffled medical observers when he had himself buried for forty days in a locked airtight chest. The great Indian Sanskrit scholar Surendra Nath Dasgupta wrote:

> Even in modern times there are many well-attested cases of yogis who can remain in this apparently lifeless condition for more than a month. I have myself seen a case where the yogi stayed in this condition for nine days.[5]

Scientists now believe that in such experiments breathing is slowed down so much that it is imperceptible. Even if no complete cessation of the breath is possible, the yogic technique of prolonged breath retention (*kumbhaka*) is still a formidable accomplishment, which challenges orthodox medical views of what is physically possible without contracting brain damage through oxygen starvation.

Breath control is a theory-laden practice, for it is bound up with the idea of various *prana* currents on the one hand and the notion of the serpent power (*kundalini-shakti*) on the other. According to a conception dating back to the Vedic Age, in conjunction with the human body the universal life force has five functional aspects:

1. *Prana*, the incoming and rising current of the life force connected with inhalation and with the heart region and the head
2. *Apana*, the descending current, associated with exhalation and with the navel and lower abdomen
3. *Udana*, the rising current located in the throat and associated with speech, eructation, and other similar functions
4. *Samana*, the midcurrent located in the abdomen and chiefly responsible for digestion
5. *Vyana*, the diffuse current pervading the entire body and functioning, even in the absence of inhalation and exhalation

The old *Chandogya-Upanishad* (II.13.6) calls these five energy currents the "gatekeepers to the heavenly world." This phrase suggests that by knowing their respective functions and achieving control over them, one can pry open the door to the inner heaven, that is, transcend the ordinary dualistic consciousness.

In addition, five subsidiary currents known as the *upapranas* are distinguished. These are thought to be responsible for such bodily functions as closing and opening the eyelids, yawning, and vomiting.

The two most important currents are *prana* and *apana*—corresponding to inhalation and exhalation respectively—because they are like pistons powering and engine. All ten currents circulate along specific pathways, often envisioned as ducts, which are called *nadis*. There are said to be no fewer than 72,000 of these arteries, which is an arbitrary figure symbolizing a great magnitude.

The Hatha-Yoga scriptures generally confine themselves to a

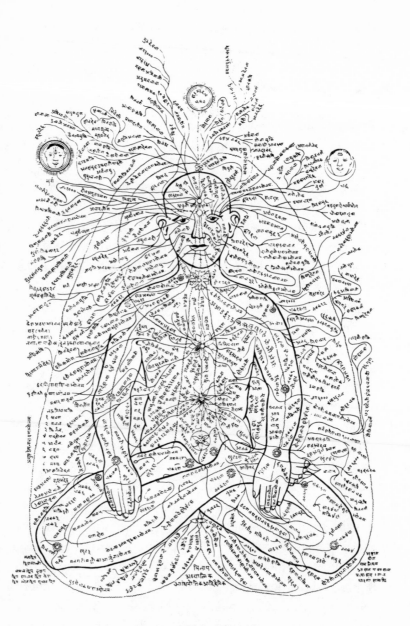

Nadis, the subtle channels
19th-century drawing from *Yoga Art* by Ajit Mookerjee
(London: Thames and Hudson)

description of twelve or fourteen principal arteries. Of these the most significant conduits are the central channel (known as the *sushumna-nadi*) and the two pathways twisting around in a helical fashion reminiscent of the DNA structure. These two winding currents are the *ida-nadi* on the left side and the *pingala-nadi* on the right side.

All *nadis* originate in the "bulb" (*kanda*) located in the lower abdomen or at the lowest energy center, the *muladhara-cakra*, and from there spread out over the entire body and beyond. *Yogins* and others with clairvoyant abilities typically describe this network of currents (*nadi-cakra*) as a treelike structure of luminous filaments.

The student who wants to practice authentic breath control and techniques for the awakening of the serpent power must accept this traditional map of the body's energetic field. To do otherwise would be to court disaster. The consequences of faulty *pranayama* practice, especially when the *kundalini* enters the wrong pathway, can be severe, including physical collapse and mental imbalance. The tribulations of Gopi Krishna, who accidentally awakened the serpent power, are well known in yogic circles in the West.[6]

The first task of breath control is to regulate, or harmonize, the various life currents in the body. The second task is to guide the life force along the central axis, the *sushumna-nadi* ("most gracious conduit"), which extends from the lowest energy center or *cakra* at the base of the spine to the energy center at the crown of the head. As the author of the *Hatha-Yoga-Pradipika* explains,

> When the life force flows through the *sushumna*, the mind becomes steady. (II.42)

This is the acknowledged method for achieving both health and ecstasy (*samadhi*) through the awakening of the serpent power, the "support of all Yoga practice," as the *Hatha-Yoga-Pradipika* (III.1) puts it. Through breath control the *yogin* energizes and harmonizes the body and thus creates a solid foundation for mental concentration and the induction of higher states of consciousness, as well as the complete transcendence of the body-mind in the moment of enlightenment.

The Eight Classical Techniques of Pranayama

The *Gheranda-Samhita* describes eight *pranayama* practices, which the *yogin* is expected to master. They are called "pots" (*kumbhaka*), which is a technical expression for breath retention. These eight techniques are as follows:

1. *Sahita-kumbhaka* ("joined pot") is a complex practice combining visualization with inhalation, retention, and exhalation in a 1:4:2 rhythm, in conjunction with the abdominal lock (*uddiyana-bandha*) just before retention of the breath.

2. *Surya-bheda-kumbhaka* ("sun-piercing pot") is performed by inhaling exclusively through the right (solar) nostril and exhaling only through the left (lunar) nostril, in conjunction with the throat lock (*jalandhara-bandha*) during breath retention.

3. *Ujjayi-kumbhaka* ("victorious pot") is executed by inhaling through both nostrils, retaining the *prana* in the nose, then drawing it further into the mouth and holding it there for as long as is comfortable by means of the throat lock.

4. *Shitali-kumbhaka* ("cooling pot") is performed by inhaling through the mouth and along the curled tongue and exhaling through both nostrils after a short period of retention.

5. *Bhastrika-kumbhaka* ("bellows pot") consists in rapid inhalation and exhalation through both nostrils, which move like bellows.

6. *Bhramari-kumbhaka* ("beelike pot") consists in prolonged breath retention after inhalation, while blocking the ears and intently listening to the various inner sounds (*nada*). The practice gets its name from the humming sound deliberately produced during inhalation and exhalation.

7. *Murccha-kumbhaka* ("swooning pot") consists in gentle breath

retention supported by the throat lock, while concentrating on the spot between the eyebrows ("third eye"), followed by slow exhalation. This practice causes a euphoric state reminiscent of fainting.

8. *Kevali-kumbhaka* ("solitary pot") is performed simply by retaining the breath for as long as possible. This technique should be done five to eight times a day, with one to sixty-four repetitions per session.

When done properly, *pranayama* has a dramatic effect on the body. The *Hatha-Yoga-Pradipika* (II.12) mentions three successive symptoms or signs. The first sign is profuse perspiration. Next the body starts to tremble. This is followed by the upward rush of the life force into the crown center, which is a process with its own characteristic symptoms. The American Sanskrit scholar Theos Bernard, who underwent a traditional training in Hatha-Yoga, witnessed these signs of successful *pranayama* practice in his own case. He wrote:

> I experienced the first stage at the very onset. After one or two rounds the perspiration began to flow freely. . . . It was several weeks before I observed the second stage, quivering, and this was at a time when I was perfecting bhastrika. First there appeared itching sensations. As I continued the practice, the sensations increased. Soon I began to feel as though bugs were crawling over my body. While I was working, my legs would suddenly shake. Later, other muscles unexpectedly contracted, and soon my whole body would shake beyond control. At this time I was told always to use the padmasana posture. This prevented the body from going into convulsions. By adhering to my schedule, these manifestations all passed away.[7]

Bernard experienced the third stage, the entrance of the life force into the central channel, during the concluding ceremony at the end of his training. It resulted in an ecstatic state that he characterized, however, as a mental experience rather than genuine *samadhi*. "It was," he observed, "a state of mind created by ceremony."[8] His teacher told him that to enjoy the experience of actual *samadhi*, Bernard would have to continue his vigorous Yoga practice until all impurities in his body-mind were removed. Unfortunately, Bernard died prematurely in an accident in the Himalayas before he could conclude his personal experiment.

Yogins pay attention to signs of progress on the way to perfection and derive encouragement and strength from them. They also respond to warning signs, for Yoga is a subtly balanced enterprise. According to the *Hatha-Yoga-Pradipika* (II.17), incorrect *pranayama* practice can cause hiccups, asthma, headache, and other ailments. Although the Sanskrit scriptures here and there refer to auspicious as well as inauspicious signs, such signs really belong to the rich oral lore of Yoga.

8

Pathways of Concentration
and Meditation

Yoga is difficult to attain by one who is undisciplined.
—Bhagavad-Gita VI.36

Withdrawing the Senses from the Outer World

The *yogins* aspire to a state of inner balance that attunes them to
the blissful Reality, or Self, throughout the day. To promote this
tranquillity and joyous participation in our true nature, they carefully
guard the senses, which are gates to the bodily fortress (*pura*). It
is through the sensory doorways that the external world constantly
impinges on the internal environment. Our senses are incessantly
bombarded with innumerable impressions that clamor for our attention. Long ago, the sages of India spoke of the sensory impressions
as poisons for the mind, since they disrupt its natural repose and
seduce it to chase after them like a butterfly drunk with the nectar
of flowers. The extent to which we are exposed today to disruptive
noise and a never-ending stream of images of all kinds is unparalleled
in history and could barely have been foreseen by the Yoga masters
of antiquity.

But the yogic principle of guarding the senses as the first direct
step in the process of inner concentration remains the same. It is as

difficult today as it was thousands of years ago. At the same time, it is just as possible as it was then. We all have an inbuilt capacity to shut out external influences from our consciousness. We do so daily in our sleep, and we can learn to do so at will while retaining full awareness. Although we have forgotten how to voluntarily abide in a state of consciousness uninterrupted by external stimuli, our deeper mind nevertheless craves to retrieve its autonomy.

In Yoga this practice is known as *pratyahara*, generally translated as sense withdrawal or sensory inhibition. This Sanskrit word is composed of the prefixes *prati* ("counter, away from") and *a* (an intensive) and the verbal root *hri* ("to pull"). It means literally "pulling away from," which describes very well the mechanism and purpose of this technique. The Sanskrit texts compare this practice to a tortoise's retracting its limbs into its shell. Another frequent metaphor is that of unruly horses that pull the chariot—the mind—aimlessly hither and thither. The *Mahabharata* epic contains these stanzas:

> The Self cannot be perceived with the senses that, disunited, scatter to and fro and are difficult to restrain for those whose self is not prepared. (XII.194.58)
>
> Clinging to that [Self], the sage should, through absorption, concentrate his mind to one point by "clenching" the host of the senses and sitting like a log.
>
> He should not perceive sound with his ear, not feel touch with his skin. He should not perceive form with his eyes and not taste tastes with his tongue.
>
> Also, the knower of Yoga should, through absorption, abstain from all smells. He should courageously reject these agitators of the group of five [senses]. (XII.195.5–7)

The problem is that, in practice, when we try *not* to hear a sound, we focus on it all the more. Therefore, instead of getting the mind not to pay attention to sensory input, the *yogin* concentrates on a selected internal object. Thus sensory inhibition and concentration go hand in hand.

To assist this process, it helps to find a quiet, harmonious place—not necessarily a sensory deprivation chamber or samadhi tank—that allows one to focus inwardly, without fear of sudden interruption. Of course, it also helps to practice all the preceding limbs of the eight-fold yogic path, which ensure a gradual simplification of one's life and a drastic reduction in the usual pressures and tensions.

Without harmonizing one's daily life through the practice of moral discipline (*yama*) and self-restraint (*niyama*), sense withdrawal is barely possible. As soon as we try to quiet our minds, we tend to think of everything under the sun. In particular, we find that all the repressed and unassimilated psychic material of the day (and of long ago) bubbles up, forcing our consciousness to seek relief by external-izing through the senses. This is a natural enough process, but it foils Yoga. We can greatly reduce the mind's tendency to externalize attention by cultivating a balanced, calm disposition at all times, not merely for a few minutes a day.

At the base of such a disposition is an attitude of dispassion (*vaira-gya*) or detachment toward material things and concerns. We can only be distracted by those sensory inputs that we, knowingly or un-knowingly, desire. Attention is highly selective and follows well-established pathways of thinking and feeling. A well-known Buddhist story tells of two monks crossing a shallow river. One monk helped a beautiful young woman across by carrying her on his back. Afterward the other monk repeatedly told him that this seemingly innocuous act of kindness was bound to poison his mind with lustful thoughts in the long run. The first monk laughingly responded that whereas he had left the young woman behind at the river, his fellow monastic was still carrying her around in his head.

Swami Nikhilananda—following the advice of Swami Viveka-nanda—offered this picturesque description of the mechanism of attention:

> We retain the impression of an object only when the mind
> is attached to it through a sense-organ. Thus we may see,

during the daytime, a thousand faces, but we remember at night only the face to which the mind felt attached. By means of pratyahara, the yogi can check the outward inclination of the mind and free it from the thraldom of the senses. The mind of the average person may be likened to a monkey which, restless by nature, has taken a deep draft of liquor, thus aggravating its restlessness, further has been stung by a scorpion, and finally has been possessed by a ghost. Just so, the naturally restless mind, after a deep dose of worldly pleasures, becomes intensely restless; it is, further, stung by jealousy, and finally possessed by the ghost of egotism.[1]

In the face of the mind's great fickleness, Swami Nikhilananda recommended that meditators simply allow the mind to gyrate until it exhausts itself. The problem with this approach is that it may take a long time for this to happen because few beginners are able to stand back sufficiently from the inner drama and allow it to run its course. Another, more demanding method is to check attention by sheer willpower—a feat of which exceedingly few people are capable for any appreciable length of time. A third approach is to gently return the roving mind to the same object of concentration, which is the method favored by Patanjali in his *Yoga-Sutra*.

Discovering the Inner World through Concentration

In his excellent book *Yoga and the Hindu Tradition*, the French scholar Jean Varenne relates the anecdote of the mathematician who, strolling through the streets of Paris, was struck by an idea.[2] He happened to find himself in front of a hansom cab. Oblivious to his surroundings, he pulled a piece of chalk out of his pocket and promptly started to develop his mathematical equations on the cab's black cloth surface. Before he could complete his calculations, however, the cab drove off, with the mathematician running after it eager to finish his task.

In Yoga the voluntary stoppage of the outgoing tendencies of the mind is called *dharana*, meaning "holding" or concentration. Patanjali defines concentration as "the binding of consciousness to a [single] place" (*Yoga-Sutra* III.1). It is clear from the commentaries on Patanjali's aphorisms that by "place" (*desha*) is meant any focal point inside the body-mind, notably the psychoenergetic centers (*cakra*) at the base of the spine, sexual organs, navel, heart, throat, forehead, and crown of the head. But the *yogin* may also focus his attention on a specific thought or image, or on a single sound or sound pattern, whether heard externally or internally. It is even possible to achieve concentration with regard to an external object, such as the flame of a candle or an icon. In each case, however, the focus must be maintained for a long time, until consciousness becomes naturally internalized.

For instance, a Yoga practitioner might recite aloud the sacred utterance SHIVO'HAM, SHIVO'HAM, SHIVO'HAM ("I am Shiva") over and over again. After several weeks or months of daily practice, this mantra will have so engrained itself upon the mind that the practitioner finds himself or herself spontaneously reciting it silently whenever the mind is not occupied with a task. Next the practitioner may wish to cultivate silent recitation, allowing the mental echo of the *mantra* to carry his or her attention to ever deeper levels of experience. In due course, the *mantra* becomes constant "background noise," regardless of whatever else the Yoga practitioner may be doing or thinking. But this "noise" is harmonizing rather than disturbing. Ultimately, the *mantra* reveals its essence, which is the nondual consciousness of Shiva, the ultimate Reality.

Another method involving concentration upon sound is known as *nada-yoga*. Here the practitioner focuses attention upon the inner sound (*nada*), for instance, in the form of the mental echo of the nasalized or hummed *m*-sound of the sacred syllable OM. In this way, the practitioner discovers ever more subtle levels of sound through the progressive ability to focus attention and shut out external stimuli.

Concentration upon various manifestations of inner light is also a powerful way of disciplining the mind. This is the orientation of the once apparently widespread but now little-known *taraka-yoga* of northern India. Swami Muktananda described his experiences with various lights of white, blue, red, and even black color in his autobiography, *Play of Consciousness.*[3]

Apart from *mantra* recitation, the most widely preferred concentration practice is visualization, in which a more or less complex mental image is gradually assembled until it achieves great vividness and is capable of holding the mind for a prolonged period of time in a state of meditation. This method has been developed into a sophisticated science in Tantrism, notably Vajrayana Buddhism, but also in Hatha-Yoga.

The *Vijnana-Bhairava*, an important scripture of Shaiva Yoga of Kashmir, describes 112 methods for concentrating the mind and bringing about the interiorization of awareness. This text employs the word *bharana* ("bearing") for the process of concentration. It recommends, among other focal points, the five voids (*shunya*) in the heart, the central channel running along the bodily axis, the sound of a musical instrument, the flow of the breath, the universe in its entirety, and even sexual pleasure or the memory of sexual pleasure (so long as it does not lead to distraction).

Whatever prop is used to focus attention, it must be employed repeatedly to serve the purpose of concentrating the mind effectively. In other words, yogic concentration must become a habit—a habit, no less, that overcomes our chronic addiction to externalizing our consciousness.

Creative Meditation

When attention remains focused for a period of time without too much effort, a noticeable change in the quality of one's consciousness spontaneously occurs. This new quality is known as *dhyana* or meditation. All the normal outside stimuli no longer disrupt one's inner state of calmness, and mental focusing comes easier and is even in some sense pleasurable. The turmoil of thoughts has died down considerably, and there is a continuity in the flow of the ideas arising in the mind. Hence Patanjali defined meditation as "the single flow of ideas in that [state of concentration]" (*Yoga-Sutra* III.2). That is, in meditation, the arising ideas are identical. Thus, if the practitioner meditates on a particular deity, the image of that deity will appear in every instant for as long as the flux of meditative attention is not broken. The *yogins* realized early on that the empirical consciousness (*citta*)—like everything else in the manifest world—is continually oscillating or blinking in and out of existence. Only the transcendental Consciousness or Awareness is absolutely stable.

Concentration and meditation represent an effort to create continuity within this discontinuity by making the successively arising ideas (*pratyaya*) similar to each other. This has the desired practical effect of focusing attention on seemingly the same object or idea, which creates a highly unified mental environment.

The inner continuum created through meditation is also highly energetic—a fact that is seldom appreciated by nonmeditators or even beginners on the meditative path. Indeed, meditation cannot deepen and give rise to ecstasy (*samadhi*) without being accompanied by an intense psychoenergetic charge. For this very reason, breath control precedes the so-called "inner limbs" (*antar-anga*) of concentration, meditation, and ecstasy. Through the practice of *pranayama*, the *yogins* supercharge their system with life force, and they also do everything in their power, including practicing celibacy, to conserve the life force in the body. Even thinking and worrying expend life energy and therefore must be checked.

Inducing the ecstatic state calls for a considerable amount of psychoenergy. What is more, this high-voltage *prana* must be properly balanced in the body and, like a laser beam, enter the central channel and travel in a flash to the topmost psychoenergetic center at the crown of the head. So long as there are obstructions in the body's energetic pathways, this process is likely to be accompanied by unpleasant and disturbing psychosomatic phenomena. Therefore, to succeed in meditation, it is crucial to strictly adhere to all the fundamental moral observances and also to undergo the obligatory purification practices. Yoga forms a cohesive system of physical, emotional, mental, and spiritual purification and integration. No aspect must be omitted, because otherwise imbalances remain, or are introduced, that can have disastrous consequences for the practitioner later.

That Yoga can be viewed as a comprehensive process of purification was clearly expressed by the Buddhist monk Buddhaghosa, who lived around 400 CE. In his *Visuddhi-Magga* (Path of Purification), a meditation manual written in the Pali language, he gave detailed information about the proper environment and conditions for practicing meditation. He also emphasized the need for moral purity as a prerequisite for concentration and meditation practice. In fact, the entire first chapter of the *Visuddhi-Magga* revolves around the nature and role of virtue on the Buddhist path.

Similar to Patanjali, Buddhaghosa defined concentration as "one-pointedness of the mind." One-pointedness (*ekaggata* in Pali; *ekagrata* in Sanskrit) is the focus of attention on a single object. Unlike Patanjali, he did not make a distinction between concentration and meditation because the two form a continuous process.

Buddhaghosa mentioned forty-two props suitable for concentration or meditation: ten *kasinas* (or bright shiny objects such as colored wheels or the elements); ten loathsome objects (that is, corpses in various stages of decay); ten ideas (such as the Buddha, the Buddhist teaching, the Buddhist community, and peace); the four sublime states (universal friendship, compassion, joy, and equanimity); the four formless states (infinite space, infinite consciousness, nothingness, and the realm beyond perception and nonperception); and the four qualities of the material elements (extension, movement, heat, and cohesion).

Virtually anything can be made into a meditative prop for the inwardly focused attention. As the practitioner's capacity for concentration increases, he or she can more and more easily apply this skill to all kinds of objects and situations. In his *Tattva-Vaisharadi* (Elucidation of Reality) commentary on the *Yoga-Sutra,* Vacaspati Mishra suggests that the *yogin* should practice concentration first upon a coarse (physical) object and only later upon a subtle (mental) object, just as an archer begins by shooting at a big target that is close by and then, as his skill improves, at a small target that is placed increasingly farther away.

After suggesting a variety of methods, Patanjali in his *Yoga-Sutra* (I.39) observes that restriction (*nirodha*) of the contents of consciousness can be accomplished by meditation "as desired" (*yatha abhimata*). It is obviously easier to focus the mind on something to which we are naturally drawn.

A traditional story illustrates this point in a humorous way. A young man called Krishna came to a sage asking for instruction in meditation. The sage recommended that he picture his namesake Lord Krishna seated on a lotus in his heart while repeating a particular *mantra.* Suddenly looking quite distraught, the young man said: "I beg your forgiveness, but my mind is on the dense side and so I am unable to follow your instructions. They are too complicated, and I won't even be able to remember them." Feeling compassion for his new student, the sage suggested an alternative: to gaze attentively at an image of Lord Krishna to the exclusion of everything else. Again the lad looked troubled. He responded: "Master, I don't think I can do this either. I would have to sit quite still *and* look at the image at the same time."

Patiently, the sage asked his student what he was most fond of. The lad's eyes lit up, and he said: "The cow in my home. I constantly think of her because of all the milk, curd, and ghee she provides."

The sage told the young man to go to the back room, sit down, and simply think of his cow to his heart's content for as long as he could. With a huge smile on his face, the lad obeyed. Three days later the simpleminded student was still sitting in the same spot. The teacher called out to him that it was time to come out and take some nourishment. The lad answered: "Moo. I am too large to fit through the door." The student had succeeded in his meditation: He had inwardly *become* his favorite cow. The sage then instructed him to change his meditation and contemplate the real nature of the cow, which is the formless but blissful ultimate Reality. The young man was able to follow his teacher's final instruction, and, moving beyond name and form, discovered the true essence of his favorite animal and of himself.

Using the Power of the Imagination

One of the traditional forms of meditation is visualization, which involves the imaginative powers of the mind. Imagination is that mental faculty that is able to form concepts or images in the absence of sensory data. As the *yogins* of India and the *magi* of Europe have known for a long time and as Carl Gustav Jung has rediscovered for Western psychology, imagination is the psyche's most powerful capacity. Unlike dreams or reveries, the yogic imaginative visualizations are consciously structured, are controlled processes, and have a specific purpose: to liberate, in psychoanalytic language, the practitioner from the clutches of the unconscious.

Broadly put, through our imagination we are able to create images, which need not necessarily be visual. These images can involve sound, touch, smell, or movement. Most people find it easiest to generate visual and auditory images, and the former can have an especially potent influence on the physical body. In most cases, however, the imagery we create tends to lack vividness and vitality. Therefore yogic practitioners, like initiates of the magical arts, spend a great deal of time strengthening their faculty of imagination. This enables them to create vivid three-dimensional images of their meditation object and hold them stably for a prolonged period of time, so that these images can have a profound and long-lasting effect on the psyche and even the body.

Visualization is particularly cultivated in Tantrism, especially the Vajrayana (Tantric) Buddhism of Tibet. Here visualization of specific deities is thought to complement and surpass the practice of the virtue perfections (*paramita*) such as generosity, patience, and compassion, as taught in the Sutras of Mahayana Buddhism. This so-called Deity Yoga (*deva-yoga*) is explained in the Buddhist Tantras as combining both wisdom (*prajna*) and method (*upaya*).

Deity Yoga is the essential practice of what is known as the Highest Yoga Tantra (*anuttara-yoga-tantra*), which proceeds in two phases. The first phase is the stage of generation (*utpatti-krama*), consisting in the creation of vivid visualizations first of a deity apart from oneself and then of oneself as identical with that deity. The second phase is the stage of completion (*nishpanna-krama*) in which the transformation achieved on the imaginative or mental level crystallizes to the point of concreteness. First one actually becomes the visualized deity and in due course realizes the deity's and one's own ultimate nature, which is the Buddha nature.

The stage of generation has two levels. On the first level, the deities are visualized together with their respective environments, known as *mandalas* ("circles"). On the second, subtle level, both deities and their environments are visualized within a tiny drop. As the practitioner progresses, his or her visualizations become increasingly detailed. The details are drawn from special manuals of instruction and a teacher's oral commentary. The deities are not so much divinities in the Hindu sense but Buddhas and transcendental Bodhisattvas. Favorite deities for visualization are the five Dhyani (Meditator) Buddhas (Vairocana, Akshobhya, Amitabha, Ratnasambhava, and Amoghasiddhi). Thus the visualizations on the path of the Highest Yoga Tantra are partly fictional and partly real. As visualization practice deepens, the practitioner becomes increasingly able to infuse his or her visualization with the reality of the actual Buddhas and Bodhisattvas—until virtual Buddhahood is accomplished.

John Blofeld explained the Tantric approach in this way:

> How visualization achieves its results is hard to convey because it is based on assumptions foreign to Western thought (although not quite unfamiliar to the Jungian school of psychology). The methods bear a more than superficial resemblance to magic arts generally dismissed as hocus-pocus. By Vajrayana adepts, however, the fundamental identity and interpenetration of all things in the universe is accepted as self-evident and the mandala (great circle of peaceful and wrathful deities) on which visualization is often based is recognized as a valid diagram of the interlocking forces which in their extended form comprise the entire universe and in their contracted form fill the mind and body of every individual being. Each of the deities with whom union is achieved has a vital correspondence with one of those forces; therefore the mind-created beings can be used to overcome all obstacles to our progress.[4]

In Deity Yoga, the intense visualizations are counterbalanced by an awareness of the ultimate void (*shunya*) of all things, including visualized beings. The *yogins* know that to reach liberation they must dissolve again the deity they have called forth in their own mind and, in that process, dissolve the ego illusion.

Practical Preparations

Apart from the factors already mentioned, several other general preparatory disciplines promote concentration and meditation. It helps to meditate in a familiar environment where interruptions are predictably minimized, engendering a feeling of safety. Also, repeated meditation in the same location sets up an energy imprint that allows the practitioner to enter the meditative state more quickly.

Most traditional authorities agree that the early morning is the best time for meditation. In India, the *yogins* typically meditate at sunrise, known as the "hour of Brahma" (*brahma-muhurta*). It is thought that the quality of the life force (*prana*) is then particularly pure and strong and more easily assimilated. But meditation at noon, sunset, and midnight is also recommended, for each time has its own distinct quality. Whatever one's preferred time for meditation, it is useful to meditate regularly and at roughly the same time.

Beginners are usually advised to sit in meditation for no more than fifteen minutes at a time, as otherwise there is a tendency to become restless or fall asleep. In that case, the mind is inclined to indulge in fantasies that have no desirable effect and merely reinforce wrong mental habits. Whenever sleep threatens to overcome a beginner, he or she may pay attention to the breath for a while before returning to the prescribed concentration technique. For this reason it is also advisable to be adequately rested for meditation. Tiredness merely invites sleep or daydreaming.

Moreover, practitioners should avoid eating and drinking shortly before meditating. Likewise they should not be overly hungry, because an empty stomach can be just as troublesome as a stomach busy with digesting food. Also, sexual activity shortly before meditation should be avoided, as it depletes the psychoenergetic centers (*cakra*).

It is best to approach each meditation session with great faith but no particular expectations, which would only limit the inner process and perhaps channel it into undesirable directions. When a student complained about not having any experiences in meditation at all, Pandit Usharbudh Arya made the following reassuring observations:

Congratulations that you are free of all these interferences! If you are looking for flashing, colorful lights, go downtown any Saturday night. If you like thundering sound, stand by any highway. Meditation is not a melodrama or a theatrical performance. The only effect you should look for is an experience of stillness, first gradual and then absolute; the relaxation of the body, silence of speech, evenness of breath, tranquility of mind and the feel of an energy force within you, the life force and the consciousness force.[5]

The importance of correct motivation in spiritual practice cannot be overemphasized. A practitioner must have high aspirations to mobilize the necessary energy for the task of self-transcendence. At the same time, those aspirations must be tempered by realism and patience. Thus it is appropriate and desirable to firmly envision the great ideal of enlightenment for oneself, but this impulse to liberation must be free from neurotic self-interest.

Obstacles and Perils on the Path of Meditation

Many of the difficulties that can be encountered on the spiritual path in general may also obstruct meditation. Foremost among them are wrong motivation and wrong attitudes or negative moods. The *Yoga-Sutra* (I.30) lists several such obstacles as part of the mental distractions (*vikshepa*): doubt, languor, heedlessness, laziness, dissipation, and erroneous views. Patanjali additionally names illness and the inability to attain or remain stable in certain stages of the yogic process as major difficulties. These, he states in aphorism I.31, can be accompanied by pain, depression, and tremor of the limbs, as well as faulty inhalation and exhalation. To these obstacles we may add anger, envy, competitiveness, ambition, self-satisfaction, lack of faith, overmeditation (causing imbalance), pretense, arrogance, and incorrect application of the procedures taught by one's teacher.

Buddhism knows of ten "corruptions" where the meditator

wrongly feels that he or she has achieved a high spiritual state, perhaps even ultimate enlightenment. Thus the practitioner may mistake the following experiences for *nirvana:* (1) the vision of bright
lights; (2) ecstatic feelings; (3) tranquillity; (4) devotional feelings;
(5) sense of heightened energy or vigor; (6) great happiness;
(7) quick and clear understanding of the transitory nature of things;
(8) equanimity in all situations; (9) heightened awareness of mind-
fulness; and (10) a tendency for inner experiences (representing a
form of subtle attachment).

These realizations are, to be sure, signposts along the way to *nirvana* ("extinction"), but they are not *nirvana* itself. That they have
been singled out in the spiritual literature shows that meditators are
prone to overinterpret their experiences. This is where a qualified
teacher can help students recognize and cut through misconceptions
and self-delusions more quickly and efficiently.

Yoga practitioners must always remember that meditation is
merely an instrument, never an end in itself. Hence they should not
get attached to it or any aspect of it but always have their vision set
on the highest goal, which is enlightenment or liberation. Also, instead of being discouraged by one's occasional failures along the
path, it is more constructive to regard them as stepping-stones to
perfection. The best protection against the various obstacles is self-
honesty accompanied by modesty, a keen awareness of one's personal
strengths and liabilities, and not least a desire to benefit other beings. Above all, Western Yoga practitioners must curb their impa-
tience and accept that enlightenment, or freedom, will not come
without appropriate discipline and that the spiritual path is likely to
be a lifelong challenge.

9
Sacred Sounds of Power: Mantras

He who utters the single syllable AUM, *remembering Me when he departs [from this life], abandoning the body—he goes to the highest goal.*

—BHAGAVAD-GITA VIII.13

Mantra-Yoga: Unification through Sound

One of the most remarkable discoveries of the ancient Indian sages was the insight—undoubtedly based on their mystical experiences—that the universe is an ocean of vibration (*spanda*). This idea was developed particularly by the philosophers of the various schools of Shaivism current in Kashmir. They also taught that vibration, or pulsation, characterizes not only the manifest world but also the Absolute, Shiva, itself. For them, the divine Reality or Being is continuously self-transforming while paradoxically at the same time transcending all movement.

This idea, like most philosophical or psychological notions of the Yoga tradition, arose as a result of personal mystical experience rather than mere intellectual speculation. In modern terms, the universal pulsation of the Absolute can be understood as a "holomovement," to use a term coined by the British theoretical physicist David Bohm. Such a movement is incomprehensible, as it does not represent mere motion in space-time. Hence most Yoga schools prefer to speak of the immovable and unchanging nature of the Divine.

Kashmir's Shaivism received a great boost among Western students through the teaching of Swami Muktananda, who attracted a large following in the 1970s and 1980s. His Siddha-Yoga is built on the theoretical foundations of the Shaiva tradition of that Himalayan country.

Understanding the vibratory nature of conditional existence is fundamental to mantric science (*mantra-vidya*), the esoteric discipline employing sound as a means of spiritual transformation and transcendence. This spiritual approach is also known as Mantra-Yoga. According to this yogic school, all perceptible sounds ultimately derive from the universal matrix of sound known as the *shabda-brahman*. This expression can be translated as "sonic Absolute." The sonic Absolute is the eternal Word embodied, for instance, in the sacred utterances of the Vedic seers and preserved down to our own time as the four Vedas. The quintessence of the Vedic revelation is the sacred monosyllable OM, which forever reverberates in the depths of the human heart and the cosmos. I will say more about it later in this chapter.

The *Maitri-Upanishad* (VI.22), a work of the pre-Christian era, declares that the sonic Absolute can be heard as the sacred sound OM in deep meditation. This subtle sound is also called *nada*, which is said to be "unstruck" (*anahata*) or uncaused. Beyond the sonic Absolute there is the nonsonic (*ashabda*) and wholly transcendental Absolute or *para-brahman*. By contemplating the sonic Absolute, which is the lower of the two modalities of the *brahman*, the *yogins* are said to reach the higher Absolute beyond all sound, the vibratory (living) Reality beyond all vibration.

Mantra-Yoga is the path leading to the undifferentiated Absolute through the vehicle of sonic vibration. It aims at unifying consciousness through the recitation and contemplation of specially empowered or numinous sounds called *mantras*. While *mantras* are almost universally employed by the various traditions of the Indian peninsula, Mantra-Yoga uses this particular technique as its principal method.

Mantra-Yoga has its roots in the archaic Vedic hymnodies and probably developed out of much older shamanic techniques of trance induction through sound. According to Mantra-Yoga, sound manifests itself at various levels of existence, ranging from the audible sound produced by air waves to the inaudible absolute vibration. The sound we can hear with our ears is the coarsest manifestation of the sonic continuum. More subtle is the sound that can be encountered only in meditation. It is said to be produced by the life energy (*prana*) circulating in the human body. There are still more subtle levels on which sound can manifest itself, requiring for its perception the organs of the various subtle envelopes (*kosha*) encasing the physical body. Thus, at one level, sound can be perceived only by the mind, while at another level it is accessible only to the higher mind or wisdom faculty, called *buddhi*.

According to the Tantric scriptures and Yoga texts influenced by Tantrism, sound has four levels of manifestation. First is the extremely subtle sound known as transcendental sound, or *parashabda*, which enters the human body at the lowest psychoenergetic center, the *muladhara-cakra* located at the base of the spine. At this stage, sound is pure potentiality. In Kashmir's Shaivism, this transcendental stage of sound is explained as pure "pulsation" (*sphuratta*), which contains the eternal seeds for all possible sounds. It is undifferentiated sonic presence—a presence that is inherent in all sounds on all levels of manifestation. In other words, even a spoken curse or blessing contains the transcendental (*para*) dimension of sound. It is identical with the self-luminous Consciousness underlying all minds or centers of awareness.

Next comes the "visible sound" (*pashyanti-shabda*), which is associated with the psychoenergetic center at the heart, or *anahata-*

cakra. At this level, sound is called visible because it is present as an eternal sound image that is as yet barely differentiated from the transcendental sound. It is fully perceivable only in the ecstatic state. From the viewpoint of the empirical (self-divided) consciousness, it represents the initial moment of cognition when there is a rudimentary awareness of sound (or any objective form) but as yet no definite knowledge or clear perception.

The sonic manifestation connected with the throat center, or *vishuddhi-cakra*, is known as middling sound (*madhyama-shabda*). At this third stage of sonic manifestation, sound is thought, the meaning or intention that goes into the subsequent audible utterance. The middling sound is present in the higher or transpersonal mind (*buddhi*).

Finally, the vibration caused by the vocal organs is called manifest sound (*vaikhari-shabda*). This is the level of language by which beings communicate in the realm of duality.

Each of these four phases of sound—also called speech (*vac*, Latin *vox*)—represents a particular level of energy that is associated with specific spiritual realizations and paranormal abilities. Some scriptures, such as the *Hamsa-Upanishad* (Secret Teaching of the Swan), speak of ten levels of manifestation of the inner sound. Models like this are primarily intended as maps for the *yogin*'s inward odyssey and can only be fully understood through actual yogic experience.

The Sixteenfold Mantra-Yoga

That Mantra-Yoga is more than mere verbal repetition is evident from the description given in the *Mantra-Yoga-Samhita* (XXXI.1ff.), indicating the ritualistic context for this yogic orientation. This relatively recent work, inspired by Tantrism, outlines a full-fledged mantric discipline comprising sixteen limbs:

1. Devotion (*bhakti*), which is worship of the Divine, can be of three kinds corresponding to the three fundamental qualities (*guna*)

of Nature, namely *tamas, rajas,* and *sattva:* (a) prescribed devotion (*vaidhi-bhakti*) consisting in ceremonial worship; (b) devotion involving attachment (*raga-atmika-bhakti*), which is tainted by egoistic motives; and (c) supreme devotion (*para-bhakti*), which is pure and yields supreme bliss.

2. Purification (*shuddhi*) relates to body, mind, direction, and location. (a) Bodily or external (*bahya*) purification by means of bathing or applying ashes to the skin causes self-rejoicing and the blessing of one's chosen deity. (b) Mental or inner (*antah*) purification is achieved through the steady cultivation of fearlessness, cheerfulness, generosity, control over the senses, study, austerity, simplicity, nonharming, truthfulness, nonattachment, peace of mind, kindness, greedlessness, patience, and so on. This creates "divine wealth," whereas pride, inconsiderateness, and other similar negative attitudes represent "demoniacal wealth." Mental purification leads to ecstasy and the vision of one's chosen deity. (c) Purification of the (four) directions, consisting mainly in facing the east or the north (at night always the north), yields power (*shakti*). (d) Purification of the location involves cleansing the ritual space with sacred cow dung or seating oneself under certain types of trees (notably the fig tree); in a teacher's home, a temple, a pilgrimage center, or a forest; by a river bank; or in other sacred places. This practice is said to increase merit and to lead to sanctity.

3. Posture (*asana*) has the purpose of stabilizing the body for meditation. It can be either the lotus posture (*padma-asana*) or the *svastika* posture. This ritual practice also involves paying attention to the type of material of which a seat is made. Suitable seats are a silken cloth (for removing diseases), a blanket (best of a red color; for attaining one's desired goals), *kusha* grass (for longevity), lion skin, tiger skin (for emancipation), and black deer skin (for attaining higher knowledge). Unsuitable seats are the bare ground (because it is painful), wood (which brings misfortune), bamboo (which causes poverty), stone (which leads to illness), straw (which leads to loss of

reputation), leaves (which cause insanity), and ordinary cloth (which leads to failure in Yoga).

4. Service to the five limbs (*panca-anga-sevana*) of the Divine consists in the daily recitation of the *Bhagavad-Gita* and the *Sahasra-Nama* (Thousand Names) of the Divine, the chanting of songs of praise, protective incantations, and heart-opening chants. By focusing attention on the Divine by means of these five ritual practices, the Yoga practitioner becomes gradually assimilated into the divine Being.

5. Conduct (*acara*), which is based on a person's innate qualities, may be of three kinds: (a) divine (*divya*) conduct, suitable for a practitioner in whom the *sattva* quality is predominant and referring to an approach that not only includes conventional renunciation but also goes beyond worldly activity; (b) left-hand (*vama*) or heroic (*vira*) conduct, best suited for a person in whom the *tamas* quality is preponderant and involving worldly activity on the foundations of nonattachment; and (c) right-hand (*dakshina*) conduct, involving renunciation on the part of a practitioner whose personality is characterized by the quality of *rajas*.

6. Concentration (*dharana*) can have an external or an internal object and must proceed on the basis of faith (*shraddha*). It leads to the experience of the deity's proximity, vision of one's chosen deity, and not least perfection in the recitation of *mantras*.

7. Service to the divine space (*divya-desha-sevana*) is the ritual consecration of one's immediate environment for the purpose of facilitating yogic practice. There are sixteen aspects of divine space, including fire, water, *linga* (sacred phallus, symbol of Shiva), the meditation seat, the sculpted image of one's chosen deity, the ashes rubbed over the body, one's navel, heart, and head.

8. Ritual of the life force (*prana-kriya*) consists of "placing" (*nyasa*) the life force, the seers (*rishi*) connected with a given *mantra*, and the fifty letters of the Sanskrit alphabet (representing as

many types of energy) into various bodily parts to create a consecrated body.

9. Seal (*mudra*) refers to numerous hand gestures used during the ritual in order to focus the mind. These gestures are thought to increase the delight of deities and lead not only to spiritual perfection but also to material success.

10. Satiation (*tarpana*) is the practice of offering libations of water to one's chosen deity, causing him or her to be delighted and therefore to favor the practitioner with blessings. When properly performed, this ritual obviates more elaborate sacrifices to the deities, ancestors, and lower spirits.

11. Invocation (*havana*) is calling upon the deity by means of *mantras* during sacrificial offerings. It leads to both extraordinary powers (*siddhi*) and prosperity.

12. Offering (*bali*) consists in making gifts of fruit and other items to one's chosen deity. The best offering, however, is said to be the gift of oneself (*atma-bali*), for it removes the ego and thus brings spiritual success. While making the external offering, the practitioner should also offer up desire, anger, and other similar negative inner states.

13. Sacrifice (*yaga*) can be either external or internal, the latter being considered superior.

14. Recitation (*japa*) can be silent or mental (*manasa*), whispered (*upamshu*), or voiced (*vacika*). Whispered recitation is ten times and mental recitation a thousand times more effective than voiced *japa*.

15. Meditation (*dhyana*) is manifold because of the great variety of possible objects of contemplation.

16. Ecstasy (*samadhi*) is called the "great condition" (*mahabhava*) wherein the mind dissolves into the Divine or the chosen deity as a manifestation of the Divine. In the ecstatic state, the meditator (*dhyatri*), the process of meditation (*dhyana*), and the object of meditation (*dhyeya*) merge to form a unitary state of being and

pure awareness in which there are no distinctions and which is suffused with bliss.

Like all forms of Yoga, Mantra-Yoga aims at overcoming the illusion of separateness through the realization of the singular Self.

Mantras: Sounds of Transformation

The Tantric scriptures offer an esoteric explanation of the word *mantra*. They relate its two syllables—the verbal root *man* and the suffix *tra*—to the words *manana* ("thinking") and *trana* ("saving"). Thus a *mantra* is a power-charged form of thought that serves as an instrument of spiritual salvation or liberation. The reason that *mantras* are liberating is that each sound is archetypal, capable of focusing the mind and thus providing access to the inaudible eternal Sound beyond all sounds, which is none other than the invisible eternal Light beyond all lights and the unchangeable Reality beyond all states of being and nonbeing. At the level of the Ultimate, sound, form, light, and all other differentiations melt away. There is only the One "without a second" (*advaita*). As the German-born Lama Anagarika Govinda explained:

> Mantras do not act on account of their own "magic" nature, but only through the mind that experiences them. They do not possess any power of their own; they are only the means for concentrating already existing forces—just as a magnifying glass, though it does not contain any heat of its own, is able to concentrate the rays of the sun and to transform their mild warmth into incandescent heat.[1]

The revelatory power of *mantras* is best illustrated by the Vedic hymns, which are collectively called *mantras* and which are the original revelation of the sacred canonical literature of Hinduism. The Vedic hymns, which were composed by seers (*rishi*), were from the beginning understood as sacred utterances. They are held to empower the mind of the reciter or listener to reproduce in him or her the original vision of which the Vedic hymns are the spoken (and now also written) embodiment.

The ancient seers employed fifteen different meters to produce the desired effect. Exacting recitation of the hymns in a ritual context was part of the archaic Yoga of Vedic times. Not surprisingly, the Vedic seers themselves thought deeply about their mantric discipline. In a well-known hymn of the *Rig-Veda* (I.164), the divine Speech (*vac*) is said to have four feet, of which three are beyond the perception of mortals. Only the seers, who in their ecstasies leave the human constitution behind, come to know the hidden aspects of divine Speech.

Even in Vedic times, the *mantra* was thought to have the power to reveal the Truth, which is the central concern of Vedic spirituality. Even in those situations in which the seers and sages used *mantras* to curse rather than bless, their Truth-revealing power is obvious. For such *mantras* were employed only against evildoers who reviled the divine order. They were administered as a corrective medicine. Their psychic charge was considerable, and therefore even those who fashioned them through one-pointed concentration had to guard themselves against possible backfiring. The seers, whom the *Rig-Veda* compares to skillful carpenters, were careful to "carve" their *mantras* well, so that these sacred utterances would not backfire on them but actually protect them. The Vedic poet-sages believed that the Truth or divine Order (*rita*) always protects those who hold it dear.

Some of the Vedic utterances were subsequently singled out as particularly potent and truth-bearing *mantras*. Foremost among them is the famous *gayatri-mantra*, which is still recited by millions of Hindus every day. In its original Vedic form it is TAT SAVITUR VARE-NYAM BHARGO DEVASYA DHIMAHI DHIYO YO NAH PRACODAYAT, "Let us contemplate the splendor of that excellent God Savitri so that He may inspire our visions." Savitri (sometimes spelled in the nominative, Savitar) is the Sun God—the sun being an ancient symbol for consciousness and illumination. In its post-Vedic form, this mantric formula generally is prefixed with OM BHUR BHUVAH SVAHAH, referring to the Divine, earth, mid-region (or astral plane), and heaven respectively. There are a great many variations of the *gayatri-mantra*, glorifying various Hindu deities.

According to the *Svacchanda-Tantra* (XI.55), there are twenty million *mantras*. Some *mantras* are longer than the *gayatri*, others are much shorter, and some consist of only a single syllable. A *mantra* that is well known even in the West is HARE RAMA HARE RAMA, RAMA RAMA HARE HARE; HARE KRISHNA HARE KRISHNA, KRISHNA KRISHNA HARE HARE. It was made popular by the International Society of Krishna Consciousness launched in 1966 by A. C. Bhaktivedanta Swami Prabhupada. This *mantra* consists of the names Hari, Rama, and Krishna, all of which refer to God Vishnu in various forms. *Hare* is the vocative case of Hari, translatable as "O Hari."

Relatively short *mantras* are OM NAMAH SHIVAYA ("OM, obeisance to Shiva"); OM NAMO NARAYANAYA ("OM, obeisance to Narayana," which is another name for Vishnu); OM MANI PADME HUM ("OM, jewel in the lotus, HUM," pronounced by the Tibetans as OM MANI PEME HUM). Other short favorite *mantras* are HARI OM (Hari being a name of God Vishnu) and RADHE GOVINDA ("O Radha and Govinda," Govinda being a name of Krishna and Radha being his divine spouse).

Also the great Vedantic maxims (*maha-vakya*) must be counted as *mantras*. They include the following utterances: AHAM BRAHMASMI ("I am the Absolute"), consisting of *aham* ("I"), *brahman* ("Absolute"), and *asmi* ("I am"); TAT TVAM ASI ("You are That"), composed of *tat* ("That"), *tvam* ("you"), and *asi* ("are"); SO'HAM ("I am He"), consisting of *sah* ("he") and *aham* ("I"). These *mantras* all affirm one's essential identity with the transcendental Reality, or Self.

Often only a deity's name is invoked in mantric fashion. Thus Swami ("Papa") Ramdas, a modern Indian saint who died in 1963, is said to have chanted RAM (the Hindi form of Rama) millions of times. God Rama is a manifestation or incarnation of Vishnu, the supreme divinity worshipped by the Vaishnavas. "Ram's name," wrote Swami Ramdas, "is most wonderful; its power is unlimited."[2] He poured his love for his chosen deity into the following hymn:

> Ram is the softness of moonlight
> Ram is the glint of stars at night
> Ram is the blaze of sun on high
> Ram is the blueness of the sky
>
> Ram is the whiteness of the cloud
> Ram is thunderous voice proud
> Ram is lightning's blinding flash
> Ram is the raining-downward dash[3]

The Sanskrit literature includes works containing nothing but a thousand names of the same divinity, all of which can be used as *mantras*. For instance, in the *Lalita-Sahasra-Nama* (Thousand Names of Lalita), the Goddess Lalita is invoked as *kundalini*, benevolent, peaceful, everlasting, formless, free from qualities, impartite, desireless, indestructible, eternally free. Similar works exist in honor of Shiva, Vishnu, Krishna, Devi, and other deities.

Often-used monosyllabic *mantras* are OM, HAM, YAM, RAM, VAM, LAM, AH, HRIM, HUM, PHAT. The first six are associated with the psychoenergetic centers (*cakra*) of the body, where they respectively represent the five elements (earth, water, fire, air, and ether) and the mind. Through *mantra* recitation, meditation, and other yogic means, these constituents of the human personality are purified until they are crystal clear, approximating the purity of the transcendental Self.

These monosyllables are also known as *bija-mantras* or "seed *mantras*" because they are the sonic seeds planted in the body-mind from which higher consciousness or awareness can sprout in a properly prepared Yoga practitioner. Such sacred germinal sounds play an important role in Tantric ritual but have been known and used since

Vedic times. They are not meaningless but are sonic representations of particular deities or other subtle realities. Thus KRIM stands for Goddess Kali, HAUM for God Shiva, HRIM for Goddess Maya, RAM for God Agni, DUM for Goddess Durga, GLAUM for God Ganesha, and SHRIM for Goddess Lakshmi. For the traditional Yoga practitioner, the world and his or her own body are first and foremost energy. That energy exists in varous states or currents, which are associated with different deities. Thus the consecrated body is considered to be a temple housing numerous deities.

The Sacred Syllable OM

The sacred syllable OM—used in Hinduism, Buddhism, and Jainism—goes back to Vedic times. It is only hinted at in the *Rig-Veda* but is explicitly mentioned in the *Shukla-Yajur-Veda* (I.1). From then on it became a stable feature of the sacred literature of Hinduism throughout the ages. It even came to be used in explaining the process of emergence from the ultimate singular Reality to the manifold empirical world. Thus the *Mantra-Yoga-Samhita* proffers this cosmological underpinning for the recitation of OM:

> Where an effect is experienced, there also is some vibration associated with it. And where there is vibration there always is, as is well known in the world, a connected sound. Similarly, creation at the beginning was a vibration of a particular kind. Then came the sound that is the auspicious humming sound (*pranava*) in the form of the syllable OM. (III.1)

The mantric OM is only a coarse approximation of a sound that the *yogin* hears in meditation. And the sound heard in meditation is only a rough approximation of the inaudible Reality for which it stands.

As Sir John Woodroffe (alias Arthur Avalon) remarked in his book *The Garland of Letters*, "This short syllable contains a whole philoso-

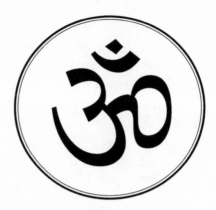

The sacred syllable OM

phy which many volumes would not suffice to state."[4] Briefly, OM is composed of the letters *a, u,* and *m.* Above the *m* is written in Sanskrit a semicircle with a dot in it. The semicircle is called "moon" (*candra*), and the dot bears the technical designation "drop" or "seed-point" (*bindu*). They indicate that the *m*-sound is to be nasalized. The crescent shape represents the unmanifest sound or *nada,* whereas the dot symbolizes the sheer concentrated potency of sound before it bursts into manifestation. Originally the crescent was written above the dot to indicate the logical priority of the *nada* over the *bindu,* but later this position came to be inverted.

The *Mandukya-Upanishad,* consisting of only twelve verses, correlates the sacred syllable OM with the four states of consciousness taught in Vedanta. This ancient text begins by stating that OM is the entire universe, past, present, and future. It analyzes the sacred syllable in its four constituent parts (*matra*): *a + u + m +* the soundless pause following the pronunciation of the other three constituents. Then the text goes on to correlate the letter *a* with the waking state, *u* with the dream state, and *m* with deep sleep. The fourth state, which is mere silence, is said to transcend the other three states. It is identical with the universal consciousness of the Self, which is neither inwardly aware nor outwardly aware but pure consciousness, incomprehensible, without distinctive mark, and nondual (*advaita*). This Fourth (*turiya* or *caturtha*) is declared to be the goal of *yogins*.

In his *Mandukya-Karika*, a celebrated commentary on the *Mandukya-Upanishad* (Secret Teachings of the Mandukas), Gaudapada promotes a special kind of Yoga based on the realization of the nondual Fourth. In his own words:

> When the mind is in [a state of unconscious] absorption (*laya*), it should be awakened; when distracted, it should be calmed again. It should be understood to be tainted, and when it has attained equilibrium, it should not be agitated [again].
>
> One should not taste the joy in that [condition of mental equilibrium] but remain unattached through wisdom. When the steadied mind [tends to become] active, one should unify it with effort.
>
> When the mind does not become absorbed [in an unconscious state] and when it also does not become distracted but is accomplished, inactive, and beyond appearances, then it is [none other than] the Absolute (*brahman*). (III.44–46)

Gaudapada explains that average *yogins* are scared of this radical yogic approach, which assumes that in reality there can be no contact with anything, since there is only the Self. This yogic orientation is known as *asparsha-yoga* or the Yoga of noncontact, which is at the heart of all Vedanta-based spirituality. It can be called a form of Jnana-Yoga.

While the practitioners of Mantra-Yoga may endorse the metaphysics of Gaudapada's Yoga in principle, they are more likely to resort to the indirect approach of unifying the mind by means of the meditative recitation of the syllable OM. This age-old *mantra* is typically chanted in such a way that a sound wave can be felt to travel from the navel to the "third eye" in the middle of the forehead. The *m*-sound is nasalized and is sounded the longest. Even when the audible vocalization has ceased, the meditator continues to follow the mental echo of the OM-sound into ever higher octaves of experience, corresponding to subtler and subtler realms of existence.

Because OM is hummed, it also is known as the *pranava*. Swami Sivananda of Rishikesh, a contemporary Yoga adept, always recommended the recitation of OM to students. "Live in OM," he would say, meaning that students should let themselves be carried by the mantric current to the hidden spiritual reality behind the sacred sound. Even the philosophically oriented Patanjali mentions in his *Yoga-Sutra* (I.27) contemplative recitation of the *pranava* as an excellent means for turning the mind inward and eliminating obstacles on the yogic path.

Mantra Initiation and Practice

Mantra-Yoga is a complex discipline, and it is impossible to cover all its aspects, never mind the numerous details of practice. However, a few pointers can be given here. First, Mantra-Yoga is an esoteric practice requiring initiation (*diksha*) by a qualified adept who knows how to fine-tune the aspirant's subtle energies so that his or her *mantra* recitation becomes fruitful. "Initiation," states the *Mantra-Yoga-Samhita* (V.2), "is the root of all recitation." Without initiation, the practitioner is unlikely to be able to energize a *mantra* to the point where it seems to come alive. This condition is known as mantric consciousness (*mantra-caitanya*) and is explained as the practitioner's awareness of the deity (*devata*) of a *mantra*. In practice, that deity is a form of energy. The *Mahanirvana-Tantra* states,

> A *mantra* is not successful for the practitioner who does not know the [inner] meaning of that *mantra* and [does not enjoy] mantric consciousness, even if he were to recite it ten million times. (III.31)

According to the *Lakshmi-Tantra* (XIII.34), the teacher who initiates a disciple into mantric practice is like a physician who correctly diagnoses the disciple's affliction and knows the correct remedy for removing it.

A duly bestowed and empowered *mantra* is further charged up through numerous repetitions. "*Mantra,*" declares the *Mantra-Yoga-Samhita* (LV.1), "does not succeed without recitation." Recitation (*japa*) is thus one of the keys to success in mantric practice. Svatma-rama Yogindra, the author of the *Hatha-Yoga-Pradipika* (IV.82ff.), outlines the stages of mantric practice as follows: First, the practitioner should block his or her ears with the fingers and focus inwardly, listening for the arising of the inner sound (*nada*). To begin with, a variety of sounds may be heard, becoming increasingly subtle. Thus the practitioner may hear sounds like the sound of the ocean, a rain cloud, a drum, a kettledrum, a conch, a bell, a horn, a flute, a lute, or a bee. He or she should continue to focus on whatever sound is attractive until the mind achieves perfect steadiness.

Contemporary practitioners of Hatha-Yoga seldom are aware that this cultivation of the inner sound, known as *nada-anusamdhana*, is the preferred meditation practice of traditional adepts of this yogic path. Svatmarama Yogindra calls the inner sound a bolt by which the unruly horse of the mind is locked within. In another striking metaphor, he compares the mind under the spell of the inner sound to a cobra that is hypnotized and rendered harmless by the melody of the snake charmer's flute. Then he writes:

> With constant cultivation of the *nada*, accumulations of sin are eliminated. [In this way], mind and life force (*marut*) definitely become absorbed in the untainted [supreme Reality]. (IV.105)

Traditionally, *mantra* recitation is said to have diverse beneficial side effects. Thus, according to the *Shiva-Purana* (I.23.25), recitation of the various *mantras* dedicated to God Shiva leads not only to spiritual liberation but also to an increase in virtue, wisdom, and even material prosperity.

Few *mantras* have a meaning as commonly understood. Rather the meaning of all *mantras* is in their function of producing a specific state of consciousness and energy. The energetic aspect of this process must not be underestimated. *Mantra* recitation—like breath control, meditation, and other yogic techniques—increases the life force of the practitioner. Then, through cultivated concentration, he or she can deploy the mantric power for spiritual but also worldly purposes. *Mantras* can and have been used to achieve material ends, both as white magic and as black magic. Their noblest application, however, is to enhance the spiritual vibrancy of the practitioner and ultimately to bring about the desired goal of freedom from the limited ego-personality. The proper purpose of *mantras*, in other words, is to tap into the potency of the Self (*atman*) so that spiritual ignorance and all karma are once and for all removed.

10
The Serpent Power: *Kundalini-Shakti*

I am the strength of the strong.
—BHAGAVAD-GITA VII.11

Gopi Krishna's Kundalini *Awakening*

> Suddenly, with a roar like that of a waterfall, I felt a stream
> of liquid light entering my brain through the spinal cord.
> . . . The illumination grew brighter and brighter, the roaring
> louder, I experienced a rocking sensation and then felt my-
> self slipping out of my body, entirely enveloped in a halo of
> light.[1]

This is how Gopi Krishna, a government official and scholar from
Kashmir, described his spontaneous *kundalini* awakening, which
overwhelmed him as he was meditating in 1937. This awakening of
the serpent power occurred after seventeen years of meditation,
when he was thirty-four years old. At first he did not know what was
happening to him, and when he finally understood, he was unable to
find expert help. Once unleashed, the *kundalini* stayed relentlessly
active, causing him considerable physical, emotional, and mental
suffering over a period of several years. He himself described his

experience as a "prolonged nightmare," which often left him incapable of working and meeting the demands of ordinary life.

On the one hand, the awakening opened up to him astounding new vistas of mystical experience; on the other hand, it caused him almost constant physical pain and inner turmoil. Several times, he came close to dying. As he put it dramatically but no doubt truthfully:

> The few brief intervals of mental elation were followed by fits of depression much more prolonged and so acute that I had to muster all my strength and will-power to keep myself from succumbing completely to their influence. I sometimes gagged my mouth to keep from crying and fled from the solitude of my room to the crowded street to prevent myself from doing some desperate act. . . . Each morning heralded for me a new kind of terror, a fresh complication in the already disordered system, a deeper fit of melancholy or more irritable condition of the mind which I had to restrain to prevent it from completely overwhelming me by keeping myself alert, usually after a completely sleepless night; and after withstanding patiently the tortures of the day, I had to prepare myself for the even worse torment of the night.[2]

Gopi Krishna's crisis was due to a premature awakening of the serpent power, the psychospiritual energy of consciousness itself. His nervous system and energetic system were quite unprepared for the onslaught of energy released by the *kundalini* process. His spiritual autobiography is a fascinating account chronicling his heroic efforts to bring this process under control. Fortunately, he succeeded in the end and was left with a permanently altered state of consciousness and a peculiarly altered body chemistry and nervous system. And yet, by his own admission, this traumatic experience did not make Gopi Krishna enlightened. "I do not claim to see God," he confessed, "but I am conscious of a Living Radiance both within and outside of myself. . . . It persists even in my dreams."[3]

From this admission, we may conclude that Gopi Krishna's *kundalini* awakening remained incomplete. According to tradition, the successful completion of the *kundalini* process coincides with enlightenment: not merely an altered state of consciousness but a new state of being marked by the permanent eclipse of the ego-personality or self by the transcendental Self.

Although Gopi Krishna's experience was atypical in many ways, it is highly instructive of certain aspects of the *kundalini* process. Sensing this truth himself, he was active in promoting *kundalini* research during the remaining years of his life. Largely thanks to his work, *kundalini* has become a household word in spiritual as well as New Age circles, though the reality behind this Sanskrit term is still rarely grasped. Today *kundalini* awakenings are grouped under the rubric of "spiritual emergence/emergency"—a crisis category that is slowly being recognized by the medical profession. In his widely read book *The Kundalini Experience*, first published in 1976, the American psychiatrist Lee Sannella argued that *kundalini* awakenings should be regarded as representing a spiritual rather than a psychiatric phenomenon, even though some of the symptoms can be found in psychiatric cases as well. He focused on what he called the physio-*kundalini*, the physiological effects of the awakened *kundalini*. He correctly argued that these side effects are by and large the result of blockages in the pathway of the serpent power. In trying to understand this process, Sannella correlated it with Itzhak Bentov's mechanistic model of bodily micromotion. Summarizing Bentov's findings, Sannella observed:

> The kundalini process is a process of physiological sensitization that can attune us to our inner and outer environments. Its effectiveness is, however, largely determined by the degree to which the individual has reawakened to the feeling dimension of his or her life. Only then can the kundalini experience be integrated.[4]

From a traditional point of view, the *kundalini* process is inherently a spiritual event. As Swami Muktananda, an accomplished adept of Siddha-Yoga, noted:

> Kundalini is a great spiritual power which cannot be detected with mechanical devices. For that reason, until now this has been a secret science. Whoever experiences it must do so with his own conscious body. He then tastes divine bliss and ecstasy.[5]

In light of these comments, what scientists may be able to study are the external repercussions of an intrinsically spiritual phenomenon. The usefulness of such research remains to be seen. Be that as it may, today psychological assistance is available for *kundalini* "victims" through the Spiritual Emergence Network (SEN) and the Kundalini Clinic, cofounded in the late 1970s by Lee Sannella and several other physicians and currently directed by psychotherapist Stuart Sovatsky. However, deep-level spiritual help for those who have accidentally or deliberately triggered the *kundalini* process is still hard to find, for only someone who has mastered this phenomenon in the laboratory of his or her own body can give effective spiritual help beyond the level of psychological counseling. In many, though by no means all, cases, psychologists and psychiatrists may be able to bring *kundalini* symptoms under control. Generally this means that they can help abort a process that has gone astray. But, unless they are advanced Yoga practitioners themselves, they cannot facilitate the awakening by correcting the process, repairing any damage that might have been done, and assisting the person in completing the natural cycle of the *kundalini* awakening.

What Is Kundalini?

The physiological symptoms that so concern people with sudden *kundalini* arousals and their consulting physicians and therapists, as indicated above, are only the disturbing side effects of a misdirected process. What, then, is the *kundalini* process from the ideal viewpoint, as specified in the Hindu literature? Before answering this question, we need to examine the word itself, which contains valuable clues to the nature of this esoteric event.

The Sanskrit noun *kundalini* is the feminine form of *kundala* meaning "ring" or "coil." It thus means "she who is coiled." This enigmatic name is an apt description of the essential quality of the *kundalini*, which, at its most abstract, is psychospiritual potential. It is power (*shakti*), conceived as the feminine or Goddess counterpart of God Shiva, who is pure Consciousness. In choosing the name *kundalini*, the Tantric authorities clearly thought of a serpent—perhaps a cobra—that, before it strikes with lightning speed, lies in tightly wound coils. Indeed, the scriptures speak of the *kundalini* serpent sleeping in the lowest psychoenergetic center at the base of the spine wound into three-and-a-half coils. They keep up this ophidian imagery when they describe the awakened *kundalini* rapidly rising upward with a hissing sound. Like a poisonous serpent, the *kundalini* also can be lethal—unless the Yoga practitioner knows how to handle it. As the *Hatha-Yoga-Pradipika* (Light on the Forceful Yoga) declares,

> The *kundalini* power, sleeping above the "bulb" (*kanda*), is
> for the liberation of *yogins* but for the bondage of fools.
> (III.107)

A more contemporary metaphor that might be helpful in explaining the *kundalini* is that of an electric generator. Most of the time, the generator is running at minimum capacity, supplying only a trickle of barely measurable energy. But when switched on full, it releases a high-voltage current with sufficient energy to cater to the needs of an entire city. Similarly, at least according to some traditions, the dormant *kundalini* is not entirely inactive either, releasing

enough energy into the human body-mind to maintain the life processes. Some schools of thought, however, deny that the *kundalini* is
involved in this low-level maintenance of the bodily functions and
credit the life force (*prana*) with this particular task. For them, the
kundalini represents purely static energy, whereas the life force is
dynamic.

In a way, it is easier to say what the *kundalini* is not than what it
is. The difficulty lies in the fact that the *kundalini*, through a spiritual force, has psychological and even physiological effects. All traditions agree, however, that it is the primordial Energy of the cosmos.
Little wonder, therefore, that the awakening of the *kundalini* should
be accompanied by a revolution in one's psychosomatic being. A
fully awakened *kundalini* is said to actually restructure the body,
leading, among other things, to perfect control over the otherwise
involuntary bodily functions, such as heartbeat, pulse, intestinal con-
tractions, and the brain's electrical activity. Beyond this, the basic
quality of one's consciousness undergoes a radical alteration, involving the much-desired shift from limited ego-bound awareness to the
transcendental Consciousness of Selfhood. Some traditionalists even
speak of the creation of a new body made of a finer substance than
the ordinary physical body. They call it "divine body" (*divya-deha*),
which corresponds to the "body of glory" in Christian Gnosticism.
It is said to be endowed with all kinds of special faculties that make
the adept appear superhuman (*atimanusha*).

Awakening the Sleeping Princess

How can the *kundalini* be aroused from its habitual slumber? The
Tantric and Hatha-Yoga scriptures are clear that a gentle kiss, as in
the fairy tale of the sleeping princess, is not enough. A more forceful
method is required to mobilize the static energy and convert it into
dynamic energy. In Hatha-Yoga, the forceful approach, various techniques are employed to accomplish this dynamization of the *kunda-*

lini. The underlying process is always the same: to focus the life force (*prana*) by means of mental concentration and controlled breathing in such a way that psychosomatic heat (called *agni*) is created. This process has occasionally been likened to the release of nuclear energy by means of continuous bombardment of protons with electrons.

Since the *kundalini* is thought to be dormant in the lowest psychoenergetic center of the body, all effort is concentrated upon that particular spot. This typically produces a measurable sensation of heat in the coccygeal area in which the *muladhara-cakra* ("root-prop center"), the resting place of the occult serpent, is located. Sometimes streamings of heat and energy are experienced, which uninformed practitioners confuse with an actual awakening of the *kundalini.* Indeed, many of the supposed *kundalini* symptoms brought to the attention of psychotherapists today are caused not by genuine *kundalini* arousals but by what are known as "pranic awakenings" (*prana-utthana*).

Occasionally, genuine *kundalini* awakenings happen spontaneously to people who do not have a spiritual practice or who, until that moment, may not even have been aware of the existence of spiritual traditions and experiences. From a yogic point of view, such spontaneous awakenings result from spiritual efforts made in a previous lifetime and represent a unique opportunity to reenter the stream of spiritual practice.

The Yoga texts emphasize, however, that few practitioners are fortunate enough to experience actual *kundalini* awakenings and that these presuppose a teacher's grace (*prasada*). In other words, they generally occur only after initiation. The amount of psychosomatic energy needed to stir the serpent power into action seems to exceed the potential of most uninitiated persons. During initiation, the adept teacher uses his or her own psychospiritual energy to trigger the process in the initiate. This is known as "descent of the power" (*shakti-pata*) and is not unlike starting a sluggish battery with the help of a fully charged battery while the engine is running. It is easy to see that the capacities of both batteries must be fairly similar, or else the weaker battery is likely to blow up. Hence a wise teacher will never transfer psychospiritual power to a pupil who is unprepared.

All Indian traditions recognize the need to ready the body's "electronic hardware"—the system of pranic pathways (*nadi*) and vortices (*cakra*)—for this eventuality. The pranic channels must be free from blockages so that the life force can flow freely through them, preparing the way for the ascent of the *kundalini* energy through the central channel along the bodily axis. Vimalananda, a contemporary adept, remarked:

> When the Kundalini begins to awaken, a tremendous rush of energy is released. Unless the guru is strong enough to control it the disciple will be overwhelmed with desires and will become strongly attached to worldly things, precisely because the chakras are still blocked. . . . When you arouse Kundalini before your mind is firmly under control, She will very likely self-identify even more strongly with your limitations, which can wreak havoc with your evolutionary progress. A good guru will close the doors to the lowest three chakras so that the Kundalini can never fall back into them.[6]

The Subtle Body

The *kundalini* process can only be understood—to the degree that it can be understood without personal experience—with reference to the structures of the subtle, energetic "sheath" enveloping the physical body. The subtle body (*sukshma-sharira*) has its own structures and functions. Its most important components are the pranic pathways, or channels, in which the life force circulates, and the concentrated energy pools known as the *cakras* (often spelled *chakras* in English).

According to the Hindu tradition, there are 72,000 pathways (themselves composed of life energy), which are the arteries of the subtle body. These *nadis* are sometimes equated with the nerves of the physical body, but this equation is incorrect. There is a certain correspondence between the *nadis* and the nervous system, but the details of that correspondence must be discovered through personal experience followed by a systematic consideration. All these pranic conduits originate in the *kanda* ("bulb") near the base of the spine or in the area of the genitals (the authorities are not in complete agreement on this).

From the viewpoint of yogic practice, only three pathways are crucial. The first is the central pathway called *sushumna-nadi* ("most gracious channel"), which runs along the axis of the body from the base of the spine to the crown. Along it are situated the major *cakras*. Twisting around it in helical fashion and crossing over at each *cakra* are the *ida-nadi* and the *pingala-nadi*, which also originate at the base of the spine, to the left and the right of the central conduit respectively. When the life force flows predominantly through the *ida* ("pale") pathway, the result is an overall cooling or calming effect. The *pingala* ("reddish") pathway, on the other hand, is associated with activity. The functions of these two channels are clearly related to the parasympathetic and the sympathetic nervous systems on the physical level and in the latter case stimulate metabolic processes. In esoteric symbolism, *ida* and *pingala* are fittingly represented by the moon and the sun respectively.

In the ordinary person, the life force ascends and descends along these two channels causing flux in the pranic field and, correspondingly, the ebb and tide of the psychosomatic states. Every ninety minutes or so, the pranic flow switches from one pathway to the other, so that it becomes weak in one *nadi* and strong in the other. In the physical body, this pattern leads to an interesting phenomenon, unacknowledged by modern medicine but easily verifiable: Depending on the predominant flow of the life force, the left or right nostril will be either more open or closed. At the time of the switch, both nostrils are equally open for a short period, indicating that the life force flows through the central channel. This is the ideal condition for meditation, and the *yogins* have a number of ways of effecting this even flow through the axial pathway. The study of this bipolar pranic process is called *svara-svarodaya*, which has been developed into an intricate science of diagnosis and health care.

The great influence of this esoteric discipline can be seen in many Yoga manuals. The much-loved Tamil adept and poet Tirumular included this statement in his *Tirumandiram*:

> If you breathe 166 units (*matra*) through the right conduit and then 166 through the left conduit, in alternation, you will live 166 years. (paraphrase of verse 729)

We must not take Tirumular literally on this point. However, his statement reiterates the traditional belief that there is an intimate relationship between controlled breathing and longevity.

The principal task of the *yogin* is to regulate the rhythmic flux of the life force in such a way that it gathers at the lower opening of the central channel and then rushes up toward the head. This process is hinted at in the word *hatha-yoga*, which is traditionally explained as the union (*yoga*) between the sun (symbolized by the syllable *ha*) and the moon (symbolized by the syllable *tha*).[7]

By repeatedly uniting the ascending and descending current of the life force and forcing it into the central channel, the *yogin* seeks to awaken the much more potent force of the *kundalini*. Running *prana* into the central conduit is simply a warming-up exercise, which clears this vitally important channel and also fans the *kundalini* fire.

In addition to circulating throughout the network of channels, the life force also piles up in certain places, which are the well-known *cakras* ("wheels"), also called *padmas* ("lotuses") from their appearance to clairvoyant sight. The practitioners of Hatha-Yoga generally work with seven major *cakras*, though some schools recognize nine, eleven, and more of these psychoenergetic focal points. Tantric Buddhism, on the other hand, employs only five *cakras*, which are connected with the five Dhyani Buddhas. The various models all have the practical purpose of mapping the *yogin*'s inward journey during meditation. So long as the awakened *kundalini* can safely be guided to the crown center, it matters little whether it is thought to traverse five or fifty *cakras*. Similarly, other details given about each psychoenergetic center must not be taken dogmatically. Their significance also lies in the practical domain where they can be verified, deeply understood, and used. Theoretical comparisons between various models may be intellectually fascinating but miss the point.

The seven principal psychoenergetic centers used in Hatha-Yoga and many Tantric schools are in ascending order:

1. *Muladhara-cakra* ("root-prop wheel"): Situated at the perineum (*yoni*) and corresponding to the sacrococcygeal nerve plexus, this center (portrayed as a lotus of four petals) is associated with the earth element, the sense of smell, and the lower limbs. It is the lower termination point of the pranic pathways and the resting place of the dormant *kundalini*.

2. *Svadhishthana-cakra* ("own-base wheel"): Located at the genitals and corresponding to the sacral plexus near the fourth lumbar vertebra, this six-petaled energy lotus is associated with the water element, the sense of taste, and the hands.

3. *Manipura-cakra* ("jewel-city wheel"): Located at the navel and corresponding to the solar plexus, this psychoenergetic whirl (depicted as a lotus of ten petals) is connected with the fire element, the sense of sight, and the digestive tract and anus.

4. *Anahata-cakra* ("wheel of the unstruck [sound]"): Situated at the heart (and corresponding to the cardiac plexus), this *cakra* is generally depicted as a blue lotus of twelve petals. The sound (*nada*) that can be heard when meditatively focusing on this psychoenergetic center (which is also known as heart lotus or *hrit-padma*) has no manifest cause and hence is called unstruck. This center is associ-

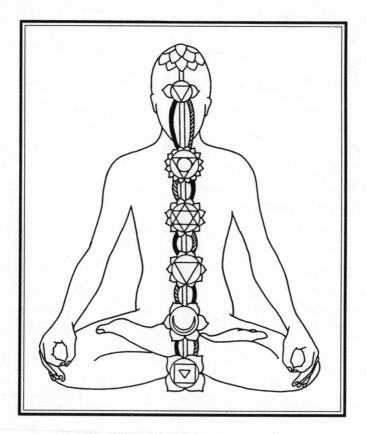

Cakras

ated with the air element, the sense of touch, and the reproductive organs.

5. *Vishuddhi-cakra* ("wheel of purity"): Also called *vishuddha-cakra* ("pure wheel"), this center is located at the throat (corresponding to the laryngeal plexus) and is depicted as a sixteen-petaled lotus. It is associated with the ether element, the sense of hearing, the skin, and the mouth.

6. *Ajna-cakra* ("command wheel"): Located in the brain core midway between the eyebrows, this center, which is also known as the third eye (or eye of Shiva), is represented as a two-petaled lotus.

It is associated with the mind (*manas*) and the sense of individuality (*ahamkara*). It derives its name from the fact that it is through this psychoenergetic center that the adept teacher contacts the disciple telepathically. Hence it is also known as *guru-cakra*.

7. *Sahasrara-cakra* ("thousand-spoked wheel"): This psychoenergetic center, located at the crown of the head, is pictured as having a thousand (*sahasra*) spokes (*ara*) or petals. It is associated with the free Consciousness transcending the brain and nervous system. The special status of this center can be seen from the fact that tradition speaks of the piercing (*bheda* or *bhedana*) of only six *cakras*. Once the *kundalini* bursts through the sixth center, the *ajna-cakra*, the full release of its energy is assured.

The Union of Shiva and Shakti

The ascent of the aroused *kundalini* power takes place in the *cakra* system. As the *kundalini* rushes upward, it activates each center in passing—a process compared to the blooming of a lotus flower. Then, as it rises higher, the center's energy is depleted and it shuts down, which is accompanied by a sensation of cold in those parts of the body from which the *kundalini* has withdrawn. In its ascent, the *kundalini* must pierce three particularly difficult places, called "knots" (*granthi*). The first is in the lowest center, the second at the navel, and the third at the throat. These points are respectively known as the *brahma-*, *vishnu-*, and *rudra-granthi*, after the three Hindu deities Brahma, Vishnu, and Rudra (one of Shiva's many names).

It should be borne in mind that this process of "piercing the six centers" (*shat-cakra-bheda*), which is fundamental to Hatha-Yoga and Tantra-Yoga, is not mechanical. Rather it occurs at the level of energy and consciousness and contains subtleties that cannot be communicated in words. Once it is inaugurated, it demonstrates its own intelligence, and so every *kundalini* awakening is a great learning experience.

Above all, the practitioner must never forget that the *kundalini* is Goddess energy. In other words, it is inherently divine; only because of this is it capable of guiding him or her to enlightenment. This fact is seldom acknowledged in Western discussions of the serpent power, which tend to approach it as if it were comparable to the energy talked about in physics. Because of the divine nature of the *kundalini,* it can, strictly speaking, be neither coerced nor controlled. Coercion and control are favorite pastimes of the ego-personality, which always seeks to predict and reshape the events of existence in order to deal with its innate insecurity and fear. In encountering the Divine, however, the ego-personality confronts the stark truth that ultimately life cannot be manipulated or controlled.

The only workable orientation in the *kundalini* process, and spiritual life in general, is the transcendence of the ego mechanism through an attitude of surrender. In other words, every *kundalini* awakening is a graceful event. This important point is emphasized throughout the traditional Yoga literature. A person may practice all the various techniques mentioned in the scriptures to facilitate such an awakening, but whether and when it will occur is dependent on transpersonal factors, notably a person's overall karma and—in Hinduism—the agency of divine grace (*prasada*). Grace enters into the equation even in Buddhism insofar as the spiritual process is thought to be always initiated by a teacher.

What happens, then, when the *kundalini* process completes itself in the mature practitioner? The divine power of consciousness rises through the axial pathway to the crown center where it leaves the body's boundaries and reunites with the ultimate Reality, called Shiva. This realization, described as the marriage between God and Goddess, is infinitely blissful, revealing to the adept his or her true nature as the ever-present Being within and behind all things.

Some traditional authorities state that the *kundalini* process is fundamental to all higher forms of spirituality, whether it is consciously activated or not and whether it is experienced as such or not. Other authorities claim that the *kundalini* arousal is a special process that is specific to Tantra-Yoga and Tantra-dependent methods such as Hatha-Yoga. They also argue that it leads to the most complete spiritual realization because the *kundalini* awakening includes the body in the process of liberation, transmuting its constituent elements in significant ways. It is true that the avowed goal of traditional Hatha-Yoga is to create a "divine body" (*divya-deha*) that is immune against the ravages of time. The very cells of this transubstantiated body are said to be conscious and capable of mind-bending feats.

Adepts like the legendary Babaji, who is said to have been alive for thousands of years and to appear only to initiates to help them in their work, are masters in whom the *kundalini* process has effected such a total restructuring of the body.[8] Reports of such adepts—called *siddhas*—are an integral part of the world of Yoga. If they sound strange to our Western ears, it is not least because we doubt the primacy of consciousness over matter. Yet, all of Yoga is firmly anchored to two basic insights. The first is the recognition—preceding modern physics by several millennia—that matter is only a low form of vibration of the same energy that exists in states of high velocity elsewhere. The second is that consciousness is not inevitably bound by matter but is inherently free. Kundalini-Yoga is a powerful method for discovering that freedom.

11

Tantra-Yoga: The Transmutation of Sexual Energy

Abandoning all norms, come to Me alone for shelter.
—BHAGAVAD-GITA XVIII.66

Defining Tantrism and Tantra-Yoga

Tantrism is the umbrella term that Western students of India's spirituality use to designate particular teachings within Hinduism and Buddhism that arose in the early centuries of the common era and were widespread by around 1000 CE. Those teachings, however, cannot be easily summarized, because Tantrism comprises a wide spectrum of beliefs and practices. To simplify, we can say that most schools of Tantrism include the following features:

1. Initiation and spiritual discipleship with a qualified adept (*guru*)
2. The belief that mind and matter are manifestations of a higher, spiritual Reality, which is our ever-present true nature
3. The belief that the spiritual Reality is not something distinct from the empirical realm of existence but inherent in it, leading to the well-known formula *nirvana* = *samsara*,

128

where *nirvana* designates the transcendental Reality and *samsara* the conditional reality (or world); the same principle is expressed in the maxim stating that the Tantric adept is capable of simultaneously realizing liberation (*mukti*) and worldly enjoyment (*bhukti*)

4. The belief in the possibility of achieving permanent enlightenment or liberation while still in the embodied state

5. The goal of achieving liberation or enlightenment by means of awakening the spiritual power called *kundalini-shakti*—dormant in the human body-mind—which is a form of the divine feminine Power (*shakti*)

6. The belief that it is possible and necessary to purify the constituent elements of the body—a practice known as *bhuta-shuddhi*—in order to create a new body of a higher vibratory order that serves the enlightened adept as a fit vehicle in the manifest realms

7. The belief that we are born many times, that this cycle is interrupted only at the moment of enlightenment, and that the chain of rebirth is determined by the moral quality of our lives through the action of karma

8. The assumption that we live at present in a dark age (*kali-yuga*) and that therefore we should avail ourselves of every possible aid on the spiritual path, including practices that are deemed detrimental by conventional moral and spiritual standards, including sexual union

9. The belief in the magical efficacy of ritual, based on the metaphysical notion that the microcosm (the human being) is a faithful reflection of the macrocosm (the universe)—"as above, so below; as within, so without"

10. An emphasis on *mantra* practice and meditation in the sense of visualization, often called *bhavana*

11. The recognition that spiritual illumination is accompanied by, or creates access to, a wide array of psychic powers

(*siddhi*), and a certain interest in the exploitation of these powers for both spiritual and material purposes

12. The understanding that sexual energy is an important reservoir of energy that should be used wisely to boost the spiritual process rather than block it through orgasmic release

Not all these features taken individually are exclusively characteristic of Tantrism, though taken together they are uniquely Tantric. Particularly the approach of the so-called left-hand schools of Tantrism to sexuality—as part of feature 8—must be deemed Tantric par excellence. It is clear from these features that Tantrism is an occult or esoteric tradition composed of arcane disciplines. Its teachings are secret or "hidden" and cannot, or at least should not, be divulged to the uninitiated. Indeed, traditionally, the Tantric initiates were sworn to secrecy. Thus, the *Kula-Arnava-Tantra*, a well-known medieval Sanskrit work on Tantrism, contains the following verse:

> You must keep this a secret and not impart it to anyone but
> a devotee and disciple; otherwise it will cause their fall. (II.6)

These words were uttered by God Shiva, who figures as the divine author of this and many other Tantras, to his celestial spouse Devi, the Goddess. Belief in the Goddess power is fundamental to Tantrism, which for this reason is also known as Shaktism. Having Shiva himself enjoin the Goddess to carefully conceal the Tantric teaching was meant to impress on students the superlative importance of such secrecy. Although this attitude has at times given rise to snobbish elitism in Tantric circles, it appears to be essentially sound. Without due moral, emotional, mental, and spiritual preparation, Tantrism can prove a dangerous trap. Its methods are potent and can backfire on those who are inadequately prepared.

Many of the Tantric teachings were never even committed to writing. They were transmitted by word of mouth from the *guru* to the duly qualified disciple. Sometimes they were whispered into the student's ear with the demand for absolute secrecy. According to some scriptures, even the gods are to be excluded from the secret knowledge of Tantrism. According to the *Kula-Arnava-Tantra:*

> Ignorant of the Truth within himself, the fool is infatuated with books, like the dull-witted shepherd who searches for a goat in the well when it is in its enclosure.
>
> Verbal knowledge is of no use for overcoming the delusions of the world, just as darkness does not cease to exist when one merely talks about a lamp. (I.96–97)

Tantra-Yoga is simply the practice of the Tantric teachings, which are supported by a comprehensive metaphysical and theoretical framework. It is not, as often thought by Western students, mere yogic sexual practice. In India, its native land, Tantra-Yoga long ago fell into disrepute because of its widespread abuse by unqualified practitioners—a danger that also strongly confronts Western adherents of Tantra-Yoga.

The practitioners of Tantrism are called *tantrikas* or *sadhakas* ("accomplishers"). The latter word is related to *sadhana* ("accomplishing"), which means Tantric practice that leads to *siddhi* ("accomplishment" or "perfection"). Those who are accomplished or perfected are the *siddhas*, often translated as "adepts." The truly great adepts are known as *maha-siddhas*, *maha* standing for "great." All these words have the same verbal root in Sanskrit, namely *sidh* ("to accomplish").

Left-Hand Tantrism

The uninformed public in both India and the Western countries confuses Tantra-Yoga with left-hand Tantrism, in which sexual union is a central ritual. Contrary to popular opinion, sex is not a universal constant of the Tantric repertoire. The left-hand path (*vama-marga*) is followed by a minority, which, because of their antinomianism, have almost always been under attack by the religious establishment and at times even suffered persecution.

Why left-hand and right-hand? In India, as in many traditionalist countries of the world, the left hand is the "taboo" hand, used for private bodily functions but not for eating or greeting. A remnant of this way of thinking survives in the English language in the Latin-derived word *sinister*, which originally meant "left." The left-hand schools of Tantrism make a point of breaking with established norms and of using taboo functions like sexuality in the service of spiritual transformation. Put differently, Tantra-Yoga uses evil (or what is conventionally thought of as evil) to overcome evil. Things that are taboo are charged with energy by the negative attention they receive. The Tantric practitioners seek to unlock that energy and convert it into positive results.

At the core of the left-hand practice is the ritual of the five prohibited things: sex (*maithuna*), consuming wine (*madya*), eating meat (*mamsa*) and fish (*matsya*), and ingesting parched grain (*mudra*), which is thought to have aphrodisiacal properties. Because all these taboo items start with the letter *m*, this ritual is known as the *panca-ma-kara* ("five *m*'s") or *panca-tattva* ("five principles").

The philosophy behind left-hand practice is this: Manifest existence is a play of the divine Energy, the Goddess. That primordial Power is particularly present in the sexual drive, which is an aspect of universal desire or *eros* (in Sanskrit *kama*). Ordinary people waste their supercharged sexual energy through orgasm. Tantric practitioners, however, harness that energy and use it to catapult themselves out of conventional reality, which is confining and associated with suffering, to awaken to the subtle realms of existence and to the ultimate Reality itself. They aspire to become immortals, who are able to participate fully and freely in the eternal play of the Goddess. With their minds firmly set on this ideal, they look upon all things as modifications of the same universal Goddess-Energy and avail themselves of any means to bring about the desired transcendence of ordinary reality.

For all Tantric practitioners, the world is not merely illusion (*maya*), as for some followers of Vedanta, but power. That power inherent in the world can be employed to both master and transcend it. Thus the world is real, not a figment of the imagination, but its reality must be properly understood. Because the world is real, a manifestation of the Divine, it need not be rejected. What must be jettisoned is the mistaken notion of the world as solid matter. Here Tantrism and modern physics meet. But whereas physics cannot and does not show us the deeper spiritual implications of its discoveries, Tantrism provides a course of action that seeks to do full justice to the energetic nature of the world (including the human body).

The Twinning Ritual

Although Tantrism includes nonritualistic approaches, which emphasize spontaneity (*sahaja*), most schools of Tantra-Yoga involve much ritual (*kriya*), particularly various forms of Goddess worship (*puja*). This is also the case with the left-hand schools, in which the central sexual practice occurs in what is known as a "wheel of worship" (*cakra-puja*), with practitioners visualizing themselves as Gods and Goddesses.

After elaborate purification rites and other preparatory practices, each participant in a *cakra-puja* randomly teams up with a partner for the duration of the ritual circle. The sexual union itself is performed according to exacting ritual standards and with great dignity and intense practice of meditative visualization.

The Sanskrit word for ritual sexual union is *maithuna*, which means literally "twinning," or "pairing." This practice is a sacred occasion that celebrates the union of God and Goddess, Shiva and Shakti, and thus the transcendence of all human experience. For the ecstatic condition of bliss marking the divine pairing is not an experience at all, since the experiencer is one with the experienced. In the state of ecstasy, the division between subject and object is left behind together with the conceptual mind and the ego-identity that could revel in that bliss.

The bliss of Being is all too often confused with a heightened state of sensory pleasure, whether or not genital orgasm is involved. While pleasure has its place in the scheme of things, it is sheer self-deception to think that it can alleviate our fundamental alienation from the cosmos, help us overcome our basic fear of death, or bring us permanent spiritual fulfillment.

Pleasure, like pain, pertains to the nervous system. Bliss belongs to an entirely different order of existence. It is not a feeling or sensation but rather that condition that prevails when all feelings and sensations as well as all thoughts have been eclipsed by the realization of sheer Being. True, ecstatic bliss is apt to register in the body, but the body—as we ordinarily experience it—is not its source. In the ecstatic condition of identity with Being, the body stands revealed as the universe itself. The physical frame is found to be not solid after all, but a vast ocean of energy in which all bodies are interconnected. Thus, bliss cannot be said to have any location or any cause.

Bliss is the everlasting "orgasm" of God and Goddess in divine embrace, beyond all concepts. It is unspeakable delight, and even to talk or write about it in such a metaphoric way amounts to a distortion of the truth. Nevertheless, language can be useful because the bliss of Being-Consciousness is our primal condition, so we have an inkling of what lies beyond words and images.

To be sure, Tantrism is neither orgiastic nor hedonistic in principle. As the *Kula-Arnava-Tantra* makes clear:

> If men could reach perfection by drinking wine, all the rogues fond of guzzling wine would achieve perfection.

If one could achieve a meritorious state merely by eating meat, all the carnivores in the world would be entitled to [such] merit.

If one could be liberated merely by enjoying a woman (*shakti*), surely all creatures in the world would be liberated by cohabiting with females. (II.117–119)

Tantra-Yoga requires something more: a profound inner reorientation that infuses all these acts with special meaning and energy.

But if Tantrism is not to be confused with hedonism, it must also not be confounded with mere asceticism. Alan Watts, one of the catalysts in the East-West dialogue, provided this insightful articulation of the Tantric modus operandi:

Ascetic and sensualist alike confuse nature and "the body" with the abstract world of separate entities. Identifying themselves with the isolated individual, they feel inwardly incomplete. The sensualist tries to compensate for his insufficiency by extracting pleasure, or completeness, from the world which appears to stand apart from him as something lacking. The ascetic, with an attitude of "sour grapes," makes a virtue of the lack. Both have failed to distinguish between pleasure and the pursuit of pleasure, between appetite or desire and the exploitation of desire, and to see that pleasure grasped is no pleasure. For pleasure is a grace and is not obedient to the commands of the will. In other words, it is brought about by the relationship between man and his world. Like mystical insight itself, it must always come unsought, which is to say that relationship can be experienced fully only by mind and senses which are open and not attempting to be clutching muscles.[1]

From Orgasm to Bliss

Tantra-Yoga, whether of the right-hand or the left-hand variety, places great store in chastity (*brahmacarya*). This time-honored discipline, common to most spiritual traditions of the world, is deemed essential to Tantric practice. It preserves and generates the vitality without which the *yogin*'s demanding inner work cannot succeed. The semen is equated with the impulse toward enlightenment, and, as the Buddhist Tantras put it, the "enlightenment mind" (*bodhi-citta*) must not be discharged. Orgasm does not lead to bliss, merely to pleasurable sensations. Even in left-hand Tantrism, the earnest practitioner must bypass orgasm.

Various techniques are recommended for this, mainly for men, since they tend to come to orgasm more quickly. Apart from great self-discipline and mastery over their bodily responses, men are advised to apply pressure at the perineum to prevent ejaculation. However, this technique can become a health hazard if it is made a habit. It is far better to avoid sexual arousal to the point where ejaculation is imminent. Besides, once the ejaculatory spasms begin, semen is released into the urethra, and the perineal trick merely forces semen into the bladder.

Some practitioners, seeking the best of both worlds, learn to control their genital functions to the point where they can suck the ejaculated semen back through the penis. This curious yogic technique is called *vajroli-mudra* and is described for instance in the *Hatha-Yoga-Pradipika* (III.83ff.), a fourteenth-century manual on Hatha-Yoga.

The merit of this exercise seems questionable, because the nervous system has already fired and thus the creative tension that could serve as a bridge to ecstasy is lost. The whole point of avoiding orgasm is to accumulate the subtle force or nervous energy called *ojas*, which is wasted the moment the nerves fire during ejaculation.

The same consideration applies to women, though some traditional authorities (notably in Chinese Taoism) claim that orgasm does not have the same depleting effect on them. The female equivalent to semen is called *rajas*, which may refer to the hormone-rich

vaginal secretions released during sexual arousal, though some authorities understand this to be the menstrual blood. In some schools
of Tantra-Yoga, men are instructed to absorb the female *rajas* into
their own bodies. But generally, the purpose of sexual intercourse—
also known as "creeper practice" (*lata-sadhana*) because of the partners' intertwining of limbs—is the circulation of energy between the
male and the female participants. Both partners use this energy to
enhance their inner identification with Shiva and Shakti.

According to the Indian scholar and Tantric initiate Brajamadhava
Bhattacharya, a person accumulates three units of *ojas* during a lifetime.[2] To attain ultimate spiritual liberation one hundred units are
required, which means that this accumulation must extend over several incarnations. Bhattacharya provides no scriptural source for this
statement, and it may well be based on oral tradition. Other schools
maintain that it is possible to reach the highest evolutionary goal in
a single lifetime. In other words, it is possible to generate sufficient
ojas through sexual abstinence and meditative practice to provide
the energetic basis for ultimate enlightenment in the span of one's
present life.

Thus, in Tantrism and Yoga, sexual moderation or even complete
celibacy is not a moral matter. Sex is not sinful and dirty. On the
contrary, the sexual drive is considered inherently divine. The reason
for recommending chastity (*brahmacarya*) is purely practical: energy
economics. The *yogins* must supercharge their bodies to be able to
tap into the universal Energy reservoir of the Shakti. To release an
arrow and hit the target, one must first pull the bowstring. The
tauter the string, the farther and surer the arrow will fly.

The reward is no less than bliss (*ananda, mahasukha*) exceeding
not only the momentary thrill of orgasm but all conceivable pleasures that the human nervous system can procure. Moreover, it is a
bliss that is not addictive like pleasure but sets us free. In the ancient

Taittiriya-Upanishad (II.8), the bliss of someone who has realized the ultimate Reality is said to be ten thousand billion billion times greater than the "bliss" of which the ordinary worldling is capable. For this supreme prize, the practitioners of Yoga willingly undergo the hardships of the heroic journey to self-understanding and ego-transcendence.

12
Self-Transcendence, Ecstasy, and Freedom

He from whom the world does not shrink and who does not shrink from the world . . . is dear to Me.

—BHAGAVAD-GITA XII.15

Releasing the Knots at the Heart

The ordinary, unenlightened individual is a peculiar perturbation in the infinite ocean of Reality. This perturbation is the product of a cognitive error that has no determinable beginning. From the limited perspective of a single human lifetime, it can be said to start with the first breath of a newborn baby. It is at that moment that the fateful erroneous identification of consciousness with a particular body begins. But its root lies in the life preceding that birth, and in the life before that, back in an elusive past.

As the child grows into an adult, this identification becomes ever more crystallized. In the end, the individual is like a spider sitting in the middle of a huge web of its own creation: all the countless beliefs, opinions, ideas, desires, hopes, aspirations, attitudes, and, not least, material belongings that stand in the service of the ego-personality and its sojourn in the world. Sri Aurobindo, modern India's greatest philosopher-sage and Yoga adept, expressed this fact as follows:

> Human nature is shot through in all its stuff with the thread
> of the ego: even when one tries to get away from it, it is in
> front or could be behind all the thoughts and actions like a
> shadow. To see that is the first step, to discern the falsity and
> absurdity of the ego-movements is the second, to discourage
> and refuse it at each step is the third—but it goes entirely
> only when one sees, experiences and lives the One in every-
> thing and equally everywhere.[1]

The ego is a counterfeit identity that experiences itself as separate
from everything else and that consequently relates to everything else
as objects that can be possessed or lost. In Sanskrit this false identity
is known as *jiva*, which can be rendered as "individual self" or "psyche" or "ego-personality." The principle of individuation is called
ahamkara ("I-maker") or *asmita* ("I-am-ness"). Its root is ignorance
(*avidya, ajnana*), and when ignorance is removed through the dawn-
ing of knowledge or wisdom, the ego vanishes, making room for the
true identity—the transcendental Self (*atman*). That Self is not confined inside any one body. It extends far beyond the skin of this body
and every other physical form. The Indian sages consider the self-
limiting identification with a particular body to be a profound delusion (*abhimana*).

The individuated consciousness seems to be connected with the
physical body at the heart. One contemporary adept has even identi-
fied the pacemaker as the specific connecting point.[2] Ever since the
time of the Vedas, the heart has been singled out as the bridge between the finite and the infinite and as a powerful focal point for
meditation. It is here, the *yogins* and sages explained, that there are
tight knots—karmically determined constrictions—that narrow the
infinite Consciousness down to the empirical mind or psyche. This
metaphor of knots was later elaborated in a three-tier model in
Hatha-Yoga, as explained in chapter 10.

In the Shaivism of Kashmir, the narrow (*alpa*) consciousness of
the unenlightened individual is labeled *atma-samkoca* or "self-

contraction." This contraction begins at the heart, at the level of feeling, namely the feeling of being a separated, isolated, and independent individual; of basic fearfulness and insecurity in the face of death and the uncertainties of life; of superiority or inferiority; of worthiness or unworthiness; of pleasurableness or painfulness, and so forth. At the level of the mind, this primal contraction manifests itself as doubt—doubt about the ultimate Reality, the invisible realms, and one's interconnectedness with all beings or one's ability to recover one's authentic nature, the Self. All this can be expressed metaphorically as so many heart knots that tie us to our born condition of ignorance, or spiritual nescience.

Through all the various means of Yoga, the *yogin* endeavors to cut these knots and free Consciousness from its apparent fetters. Its bondage is indeed only apparent—though very real for the unenlightened person who is suffering from the karmic effects of this self-limitation—because Consciousness, which is singular, is inherently free. "Freed from the knots of the heart," declares the *Mundaka-Upanishad* (III.2.9), "he becomes immortal." It would be more correct to say that when the delusion of identification with the body has ceased, one becomes what one has always been: the same all-pervasive Reality. I will say more about the curious paradox associated with enlightenment in the next chapter.

Ecstasy: When the Mind Implodes

Although the liberating wisdom always arises spontaneously and completely, for most aspirants there seems to be a path of progressive understanding or deepening of this primordial intuition. This process contains numerous "trial runs" in which practitioners disidentify from particular aspects of the ego-personality, gradually refining their self-perception. They become increasingly sensitive to all labels of *me, my,* and *mine,* recognizing them to be artificial constructs that impose severe limits on consciousness. With that sensitivity comes, through steady yogic practice, the ability to let go of all that stands exposed as part of the false self-image.

On that journey of growth, those moments involving the temporary eclipse of the ego form important landmarks for the *yogin*. These are the various states of ecstasy (*samadhi*) that can blossom through the agency of meditation or that may overwhelm the practitioner suddenly during the performance of rituals or in the midst of everyday activities.

The Sanskrit term *samadhi* is composed of the prefixes *sam* (the Latin *com-*) and *a* and *dhi* (derived from the verbal root *dha* meaning "to place" or "to put"). It thus means something like "that which is placed or put together." What is placed together in *samadhi* is the subject and the object, which in fact merge. Vidyaranya's *Pancadashi* (Fifteen [Chapters]), a celebrated Vedanta work, gives the following explanation:

> By gradually abandoning [the distinction between] meditator and meditation, the object's sphere alone [shines forth in consciousness], and consciousness resembles a lamp in a windless [place]—that is designated as ecstasy. (I.55)

The word *ecstasy* means "standing outside (oneself)," that is, transcending the ego-self. This implies, however, that one stands within one's true Self, the *atman* or the *purusha*, as it is called in Classical Yoga. Therefore some scholars prefer to translate *samadhi* as "enstasy." Here, the more familiar *ecstasy* is used, which is not wrong, providing it is understood that this state is not one of emotional exuberance. As I described this elevated condition elsewhere:

> We become, in consciousness, the bird we contemplate; we become the tree in which the sap circulates and which stretches its ramified crown toward the invigorating sun; we become the solar disk whose vivifying energies pour over the planets of our galaxy; we become the universe in its grand

immensity and pulsating fullness. We may even become one with the tranquil center in the depth of our own being, or unite with the all-comprising wholeness of the supreme Being. On whatever level such ontic identification takes place, it always presupposes the abolition of the ordinary space-time continuum and the experience of the eternal Now.[3]

In ecstasy, identification occurs with whatever object the mind was holding during the preceding meditation. At a higher level, however, that object is experienced or realized as nonseparate from all other objects. This type of unitive realization bears the technical designation *samprajnata-samadhi* or ecstasy connected with a conscious content. In Vedanta, the term *savikalpa-samadhi*, which means ecstasy with ideation (*vikalpa*), is applied to the same condition.

This form of *samadhi* yields knowledge or understanding (*prajna*) that is not derived from the senses. The ego-personality is temporarily attenuated, but it is not yet completely transcended. Although there is a radical shift in consciousness—fusing the experiencing subject with the object of meditation—the structures in the unconscious (or, as the Yoga authorities prefer, the depth mind) remain largely intact. Thus this genre of *samadhi* is not itself liberating or enlightening. That function belongs to the *asamprajnata-samadhi*, or (in Vedantic terminology) the *nirvikalpa-samadhi*, in which no ideation takes place. Here the unconscious or depth mind is profoundly restructured. In fact, if the state is maintained for a sufficient length of time, it will lead to a meltdown of the hard egoistic core, which coincides with the full reidentification with the Self (*atman*) in the moment of liberation.

The *Yoga-Sutra* contains a carefully worked out framework for classifying the various levels or degrees of ecstasy. At the lowest level, which Patanjali calls *vitarka-samadhi*, the ecstatic identification with a coarse (*sthula*) object is accompanied by spontaneous mental activity labeled *vitarka* or "cogitation." The next level is marked by the absence of this kind of mentation and is therefore styled *nirvitarka-samadhi*. This is followed by *savicara-samadhi*, or ecstatic identification with a subtle (*sukshma*) object, accompanied by mental activity, which bears the technical designation of *vicara* or "reflection." The next higher level is characterized by the absence of this type of mentation and is called *nirvicara-samadhi*.

To these four types some ancient Yoga authorities—such as Vacaspati Mishra in his *Tattva-Vaisharadi*—add the following four: *sananda-, nirananda-, sasmita-,* and *nirasmita-samadhi*, or ecstasy with bliss (*ananda*), without (or rather beyond) bliss, with I-am-ness (*asmita*), and without (or beyond) I-am-ness respectively. These four or eight types are technically referred to as coincidences (*samapatti*) because they all imply an experiential convergence of the meditator, meditated object, and process of meditation. The contemplated object is progressively more subtle.

Following is a practical example of how the ecstatic process might unfold in a *yogin* who selected the image of his chosen deity (*ishta-devata*)—let us say Shiva, the Lord of Yoga—as a prop for meditation. At first the *yogin* creates a vivid mental image of Shiva, sporting a third eye in the middle of his forehead, long matted hair, and large earrings, with his body smeared with ashes, holding a trident, seated on a tiger skin, and with a multiheaded serpent protecting his back. As the meditation deepens, the practitioner increasingly loses his conventional ego-sense and more and more identifies with Shiva. Then there is a sudden shift, and he *is* the deity. The practitioner feels utterly peaceful, powerful, extending far beyond the boundaries of the physical body. At first, various ideas (*vitarka*) flash forth in this sublime state: "As Shiva, I bless the entire universe." "I am of infinite extension." "There is no one outside of me." "I am the source of all creation." The practitioner has no awareness of time, and the space in which he finds himself is infinite, luminous, and sheer consciousness.

Then the practitioner reaches an even deeper stillness. No further thoughts arise. This is *nirvitarka-samadhi*.

Next the *yogin's* mental image of himself as Shiva—with all the characteristics specified by traditional iconography—begins to fade. But his sense of being the deity is augmented. He now is aware of himself as Shiva on more subtle dimensions that carry a vast energetic charge. When this state is interspersed with spontaneously arising ideas similar to those mentioned above, it is called *savicara-samadhi*. Unlike ordinary thoughts during meditation, these ideas do not disturb the ecstatic process.

As this state deepens, the few ideas that present themselves to the ecstatic consciousness become fewer still until a condition of total cessation of such reflections (*vicara*) is reached. This is *nirvicara-samadhi*.

At the peak of this motionless state a superlative clarity is established, which the Yoga authorities compare to the autumnal sky, which is spectacularly clear in Northern India. The Sanskrit word for "autumn" is *vaisharadi*, and this ecstatic level of consciousness is therefore called *nirvicara-vaisharadya*.

At a still deeper level, if we follow Vacaspati Mishra's model, the only content of the ecstatic consciousness is overwhelming bliss. In due course a deep calm is reached within this highly energetic state. These two phases of the ecstatic process are *sasmita-* and *nirasmita-samadhi* respectively.

Finally, only the sense of being present as Shiva remains. This sense, which is a form of ideation (*pratyaya*), also must be transcended. When this is accomplished, the practitioner (as Shiva) loses all awareness of being an individuality, though without becoming totally unconscious, of course.

At this point, the ecstatic consciousness is so rarefied that a further and still more radical shift may occur. Now the practitioner

leaves the conditional levels of existence (Nature's realms) alto-
gether and simply abides in the singular Self. This is *asamprajnata-
samadhi*, which is a state of supraconscious existence that cannot be
further elucidated. Here the very seeds that sprout into ordinary
forms of awareness are burned to cinders.

The American writer Joseph Chilton Pearce, whose spiritual life
was greatly influenced by Swami Muktananda, described the following illuminating experience:

> During an intensive one weekend in June of 1979, I dropped
> (actually I felt I had been forcibly pushed) into a deep medi-
> tation from which I immediately emerged. I "woke up,"
> more or less, but my brain didn't; my body didn't; the world
> didn't. It was given me to awake as a single point of clarity.
> This clarity was *me*, a *me* I had always been. . . . This me-
> awareness was complete and perfect beyond description. I
> was absolutely *me*, but had no name, no history, no body,
> space, time, or such. I was totally rich and perfect, nothing
> was lacking, although there *was* nothing.[4]

To unprepared individuals, this state appears as a terrifying void
from which they instinctively recoil. They fear going insane and
being swallowed up by it, which is exactly what happens: The ego-
identity is demolished or eclipsed and the mind disintegrates, at
least for the duration of that ecstatic state. To step deliberately across
the threshold into this realization of perfect nonduality would require greater courage than the ordinary person could ever hope to
summon. It would require an act of desperation. When the transition occurs, it has an intrinsic inevitability to it, which psycho-
logically translates into the momentary heroic capacity for total
surrender of everything one is or represents.

This state cannot be described because it has no content. There is
no body-mind present to provide criteria for differentiation. Yet it
does have a specific function: to reverse the outgoing tendency of

the psyche. The supraconscious ecstasy has the power to undo the game of attention by unhooking consciousness from the ego-identity. It establishes the new habit of identifying with the Self, one's true nature.

But for this new habit to grow sufficiently strong to countermand the false ego-identity and the body-mind's innate tendency toward externalization, the *yogin* must cultivate *asamprajnata-samadhi*. Having stepped through the looking glass once, he or she can do so again—and with growing ease. Then the habit of identifying with the finite body, mind, or belongings becomes progressively weaker, and the Self's benign reality makes itself felt more and more strongly in the *yogin*'s life.

When Pearce emerged from his supraconscious ecstasy, he found himself donning his ego-personality as one would an old jacket. "I had then all sorts of 'things'," he recalls, "and had lost everything."[5] If Pearce's experience was genuinely *asamprajnata-samadhi*, he had undoubtedly attained it through the grace of Swami Muktananda, who, as an adept of Kundalini-Yoga, was quite capable of initiating others into the secrets of nondual consciousness in this way. He is, in fact, known to have done so with many other students.

But, without question, exceedingly few were able to reenter that state under their own power. Ordinary consciousness thriving on the sense of duality is a tenacious habit. This habit is gradually undermined through the practice of supraconscious ecstasy. More and more, the *yogin* is pulled into *asamprajnata-samadhi*. At a certain point, he or she simply drops the body, having lost every shred of attachment to the finite world. The *yogin* now lives as the eternal bodiless Self in all beings. This is the condition of disembodied liberation (*videha-mukti*).

Sahaja-Samadhi: Perfect Spontaneity as a Way of Life

The Indian traditions also know of another route to liberation. Self-realization need not complete itself with the demise of the body. Freedom and embodiment are not incompatible. This second possibility of authentic spiritual existence is epitomized in what is known as *sahaja-samadhi.*

Samprajnata-samadhi could be described as a special state of mind in which the subject-object polarity of the ordinary waking consciousness is momentarily lifted through total identification with the object of contemplation. By contrast, *asamprajnata-samadhi* is not so much a state of mind as the temporary transcendence of the brain-dependent mind and ego-sense through the complete recovery of one's true identity, the Self. However, *asamprajnata-samadhi* does not remove all at once the preconditions for the renewed arising of the ego-identity and its associated mental activity. While the Self is genuinely realized in this rare state, that realization does not descend into the body, into the waking consciousness. The moment the *yogin* comes out of this transconceptual ecstasy, the fateful process of identifying with a particular body and mind resumes operation.

Therefore some radically nondualist schools of Vedanta deny that *nirvikalpa-samadhi* (corresponding to *asamprajnata-samadhi*) is liberating, and they consider the effort to gain or regain it wasted. This position is expressed, for instance, in the *Tripura-Rahasya* (Tripura's Secret), which was one of Ramana Maharshi's favorite texts, because it best expressed his own extraordinary state. It contains the charming story of Prince Hemacuda and Princess Hemalekha, which is meant to illustrate that liberation cannot be produced even by a hundred ecstasies. Either it is the case or it is not.

One day, so the story goes, Prince Hemacuda was surprised by a storm while hunting in the forest. He chanced upon a mountain hermitage and asked for shelter. The radiantly beautiful daughter of the reclusive sage bid him welcome, and the prince promptly fell in love with Hemalekha. With her father's permission, the two got married. While Hemalekha proved a kind and attentive wife, she did not share her husband's amorous passion or zest for life but always presented a serene and somehwat indifferent demeanor.

When confronted by the frustrated prince, Hemalekha explained that she was searching for lasting happiness and she begged her husband to help her find it. At first Prince Hemacuda dismissed his wife's explanation as silly, but when she cleverly countered all his pat answers he soon found himself in a profound dialogue with her. As a result, the prince was himself thrown into an existential crisis and ended up locking himself into his chambers to meditate and realize the Self.

Before long, he acquired great skill in meditation and finally entered the state of *nirvikalpa-samadhi*. When Hemalekha came to see him during one of his few periods of physical awareness, he announced to her that he had realized perfect happiness. But again the lovely princess quietly undermined his position with her penetrating wisdom. She argued that if he had to close his eyes and withdraw his awareness from the body in order to be blissful, he could not possibly have realized the Self and become completely liberated. She convinced him that the Self was not exclusively within himself but both inside and outside. As a result of her teaching, the prince attained true enlightenment. Of course, he also realized with gratitude that all along his wife had been enjoying the liberated condition and had been coaching him with her questions and arguments. Thenceforth the couple lived and ruled the kingdom happily ever after—in the state of *sahaja-samadhi* or spontaneous ecstasy.

The word *sahaja* means literally "together born," referring to the fact that in this condition the previously antithetical poles of liberation (*mukti*) and world experience (*bhukti*) are brought together in harmony. The *sahaja-yogin* permanently realizes the Self in all things. Such a *yogin* *is* the Self—irrevocably and without the least trace of duality. The *Ashtavakra-Gita* (Ashtavakra's Song) contains the following verses put in the mouth of Janaka, who realized the Self through the grace of his teacher, Ashtavakra:

Ah! I am the untainted, tranquil Consciousness beyond Nature (*prakriti*). For such a long time I was bewildered by delusion.

As the One I illumine this body and the world. Hence this entire world is mine, or indeed, nothing is. (II.1–2)

As waves, foam, and bubbles are not distinct from water, similarly the world, coming from the Self, is not distinct from the Self. (II.4)

Ah! I experience no duality even in a crowd, feeling as though I were in a forest. Where should I find pleasure? (II.21)

Wonderful! In Me, an infinite ocean, individuals like waves spontaneously arise, clash, play, and enter [each other]. (II.22)

Just as cloth when examined is only thread, similarly the world when examined is merely the Self.

Just as sugar made from the juice of sugarcane is permeated by that [juice], similarly the universe created in Me is completely permeated by Me. (II.5–6)

Ah! Adoration to Myself! Even though I am embodied I am the One who neither comes nor goes anywhere but exists [forever] permeating the world. (II.12)

Neither bondage nor liberation [apply] to Me. Lacking support, the delusion has ceased. Ah! Although the world abides in Me, it does not in reality abide in Me! (II.18)

Swami Rama Tirtha, an adept of Jnana-Yoga who died in 1906, composed these lines in the Urdu language, which express the *sahaja* state perfectly:

Wherever I look, I see only You.
I do not need to seek You;

I meet Your splendour in every street.
At every moment
You are present before me, face to face.

. . . .

Wherever a person goes
It is You alone who confront him.
Every home is Your home,
O You who have no home.

. . . .

Your special home on earth
Is the hearts of the righteous.
Having come to that home
After wandering hither and thither,
Now, wherever I look, I see only You.[6]

This perpetual *samadhi* cannot be interrupted by changes in the brain's chemistry, sleep, adversity, disease, aging, or even physical death. It is also known as liberation while still alive (*jivan-mukti*). From the point of view of the unenlightened mind, this supreme condition represents the ultimate paradox. From the perspective of the ultimate enlightenment, however, there is no puzzle at all but only ever-present Consciousness, which is inherently blissful and free. As the *Mahanirvana-Tantra* declares:

> That which is pure Existence, unqualified, beyond the scope of speech and mind, which is the essential true Lustre in the untrue triple world is called *brahman* (or *atman*).
>
> That [Reality] is to be known by the *yogas*[7] of ecstasy [who apply their] equal vision to everything and who are beyond doubt and without the illusion of [being] an embodied self (*deha-atman*). (III.7–8)

Gerald Heard, an early spokesman for the nondualist metaphysics of Vedanta, commented on the distinction between *nirvikalpa-samadhi* and perpetual spontaneous ecstasy as follows:

What has happened has been that the body has been left behind as the consciousness hastened on to face up fully to Reality—as a man may think so fast that words fail. But once Reality is confronted, and can be endured, then the body can and does draw up along side. Though at first shocked . . . the body can now take part in the new efficiency, in the complete allaying of conflict and in perfect functioning.

Then, as all authorities note, rapture ends, dissociation is over. The body, which had been strained—maybe unavoidably—then becomes a benefiting partner in the new life and has, in consequence, powers of endurance unknown to lower states of consciousness and vitality. Sleep is immensely reduced and so is food intake, while intense exertion can be undertaken without fatigue. . . . Every function is a process of contact and communion with utter Reality. The Temporal has become the Eternal.[8]

The British writer and sage Paul Brunton characterized the contrast between spontaneous ecstasy and other, lower forms of ecstatic merging as the difference between true philosophy and mysticism. For him, the true philosopher is the sage who, having realized the One, does not shrink back from the many. In his own words:

The materialist sees plurality alone and sees superficially. The mystic in his deepest contemplation sees Spirit (or Mind alone) without seeing Plurality, and sees incompletely. The philosopher sees both Mind and its manifold world-images as essentially the same and sees rightly and fully.[9]

And:

All yoga and mystic methods, as well as certain religious practices, although of the highest value as preliminary disciplines, are not the ultimate ends in themselves. If one has sufficient sharpness of mind—that is, sustained concentration on abstract themes—and sufficient freedom from any kind of egoistic preconception whatever, one can instantly grasp the truth and realize it. But who has that? Hence, these various methods of developing ourselves, these yogas, have been prescribed to assist us. Their practice takes a long time, it is true, but the actual realization is a matter of a moment.[10]

The effortless *sahaja-samadhi* is the very foundation of the life of the philosopher, in Brunton's sense of the term. Upon realization of the Self not only as one's innermost subjective core but also as the essence of all objectively present things, the spiritual journey is complete. Henceforth the enlightened being spontaneously participates in the unfolding drama of the world while eternally standing still as the supreme witnessing Consciousness. There is no one to fear, hate, envy, compete against, or conquer. Whatever happens, happens in the fullness of Being, which is single, eternal, and omnipresent.

13

Yoga in the Modern World

This individual (purusha) *is of the nature of faith.
As his faith, so is he.*

—BHAGAVAD-GITA XVII.3

Can a tradition that originated five thousand years ago possibly be relevant today? This question is legitimate enough. Over the past two centuries, we have seen the erosion of traditional religious beliefs, values, and practices in Europe and America and increasingly also in other parts of the world. Religion has been systematically demythologized, and many of its symbols have been deprived of their power. In the nineteenth century, the German philosopher Friedrich Nietzsche boldly voiced the prevalent sentiment among the educated classes when he declared that God was dead. Since then, secular humanism—propped up by scientific materialism—has unsuccessfully tried to fill the void created by this onslaught on traditional mores and religious creeds.

Today we live in a fragmented world that has given rise to widespread uncertainty, confusion, and hopelessness. Ours is a society of broken marriages, dysfunctional families, mounting crime, international terrorism, unmanageable metropolitan environments, drug abuse, a growing disparity between the poor and the rich, world hunger, an unchecked population explosion, environmental pollution, and the continuing threat of nuclear devastation at the hand of fanatics.

The problems we are facing individually and collectively seem insurmountable. Our local and national governments are faltering, and individuals feel a sense of powerlessness in the face of today's formidable challenges. All this amounts to a great deal of suffering and unhappiness for billions of people. Those who refuse to seek deceptive shelter in some form of religious or secular fundamentalism are understandably hungry for deeper meaning in their lives.

There is a small but growing group of people who, unconvinced by either humanistic secularism or religious fundamentalism, sense that there must be a third option that can lead them out of their disorientation and despair. They intuit that there is a living stream of knowledge and wisdom that, throughout the ages, has tended to flow underground, out of the sight of ordinary folk. And they are willing to explore unorthodox avenues to find satisfying answers to their many questions.

Among this group of seekers are those who have discovered the abundant tradition of Yoga. Why should Yoga be appealing to them when they, for the most part, have rejected their own religious traditions? The reason is the same one that is also responsible for attracting tens of thousands of Westerners to Japanese Zen, Buddhism, Tantrism, Sufism, Shamanism, and other spiritual traditions: the prospect of personal experience that gives access to the hidden dimension of existence, whether it is called Higher Self, Nirvana, God, Goddess, Truth, Reality, or Spirit. Yoga holds out the promise of inner peace, strength, clarity, certainty, wisdom, fulfillment, love, compassion, and ultimately Self-realization.

Because it is such a rich, variegated tradition, Yoga holds appeal for a wide range of people with many different temperaments and aptitudes. Everyone can discover a suitable approach within this ramified tradition. It caters to many levels of interest. However, this intrinsic versatility has occasioned misconception and misrepresentations as well. Thus, in the West, Yoga is frequently reduced to fitness training bereft of any reference to its original spiritual purpose. While such reductionistic Yoga practice may prove helpful to some people in maintaining or restoring their physical health, it must not be mistaken for authentic Yoga. It would be best to give it a different name so as not to mislead anyone, but this is unlikely to happen. At the same time, positive results from the physical exercises, however much they may be stripped of their spiritual content, can lead to a deeper interest in Yoga.

When the great psychologist Carl Gustav Jung summarily pronounced Yoga to be unsuitable north of the Tropic of Cancer, he was simply mistaken. He rightly affirmed that "nothing ought to be forced on the unconscious" but wrongly asserted this to be the case with the yogic method.[1] His own preferred procedure was what he called "active imagination," consisting in disabling consciousness to some extent to allow the unconscious to bubble up so that it could be inspected and understood. He did not think that focusing the conscious mind in yogic fashion could yield clarity of understanding or prove otherwise beneficial to Westerners.

Curiously, Jung considered Yoga to be "one of the greatest things the human mind has ever created," yet he failed to comprehend yogic psychology, which is astonishingly sophisticated.[2] According to Yoga, we can never escape the influence of the unconscious by mere intellectual understanding of its contents. Hence the yogic method aims at transcending the unconscious by directly purifying or transmuting it through the higher states of ecstatic merging. Only in this way can the unconscious as a powerful energetic system be dismantled. As the Jungian-trained British psychiatrist Hans Jacobs pointed out, Jung could not conceive of consciousness apart from the ego.[3] Thus for him the various states of *samadhi* were all forms of unconsciousness. This view is vehemently contradicted by the entire yogic tradition as well as by the other great spiritual traditions of the world.

The psychological difficulties hinted at by Jung are real enough. Many practitioners—even in India—succumb to, rather than transcend, the phantasms of the unconscious. Sadly, it also is true that many Western Yoga enthusiasts relate wrongly—narcissistically—to the Yoga tradition. But these failings say nothing about either the value of Yoga or its applicability in a modern context.

As a spiritual discipline, Yoga has universal validity. It is a practical approach to self-understanding, self-transcendence, self-transformation, and Self-realization. Although it has grown out of the Indian cultural experience and was developed in close association with Vedic and non-Vedic religious life, in its highest purpose and most refined articulation, it is equally meaningful and efficient outside of India.

The question is whether we, blinded by the apparent technological success of our materialistic civilization and troubled by its moral failure, can see clearly enough Yoga's unique contribution to our understanding of the human condition. The more we can comprehend and appreciate the pristine spiritual message of the great masters of Yoga, the more likely we will find its psychotechnology useful and astonishingly inventive.

The yogic method is beyond reproach. It springs from practical experimentation, invites and even demands practical testing, and stands vindicated through personal experimentation. Lack of success on the yogic path is caused not by any shortcoming of Yoga itself but always by a person's failure to meet the necessary criteria or follow the procedures correctly. Integral aspects of the yogic method are initiation by a qualified teacher, transmission of the esoteric knowledge (most of which cannot be found in books), and the wise counsel of an advanced practitioner during the inevitable moments of crisis.

To be sure, not everyone is cut out for a traditional yogic training under an adept teacher. Even in India, Yoga's homeland, many were called but few were chosen, as the Sanskrit scriptures readily admit. As Lord Krishna, an incarnation of the Divine, expresses it in the *Bhagavad-Gita*:

> Among thousands of men scarcely one strives for perfection.
> Even among the striving adepts scarcely one knows Me truly.
> (VII.3)

Fortunately, the Yoga tradition is embracing. It caters not only to the rare individual who is capable of practicing with the utmost intensity but also to the neophyte who is still plagued by doubts, fickleness, lack of determination, and wrong views. Yoga is like a patient mother nurturing anyone who is willing to make even the humblest gesture of commitment to the spiritual path.

It is absolutely necessary, though, to safeguard Yoga against usurpation by the consumerist mentality with which our modern culture seems to approach everything. Yoga was never intended for easy consumption, and promises of quick fixes or even illumination over a weekend are blatantly ridiculous. The fact is that we get out of Yoga (or any other spiritual tradition) what we put into it. If our motivation is misguided or weak, we must not hope for too much. If we mistake Yoga for fitness training, we will, given the right program, undoubtedly become fit. But we will also have missed the true power of Yoga. On the other hand, if we approach Yoga with high expectations but little inclination to take the practical steps for realizing them, we will merely frustrate ourselves.

Before we can hope to succeed in Yoga, we must first have a clear understanding of what it is. Therefore, study is essential. It has always been an integral part of the yogic path. But given the fact that nothing in our culture prepares us for an encounter with genuine Yoga, we must be all the more alert and take every opportunity to delve into the original scriptures of Yoga or learn directly from adept teachers.

Because our culture indulges much childish and adolescent think-ing and behavior in adults, we tend to have conflicting feelings about authority of any kind. Also, in recent years, there have been many reported cases of *gurus* abusing their charismatic power. Not surpris-ingly, the traditional teacher-discipleship has come under severe at-tack, particularly by the mass media, which thrive on sensationalism and feed the emotional immaturity of the consumer. In an earlier book, entitled *Holy Madness*, I examined in some detail the issues involved and therefore will refrain from going over the same ground here. I stand by what I said then: As with any highly specialized field of knowledge, we need guidance in our spiritual practice. A mature individual will feel no conflict about learning from a master in a given field. In the spiritual domain, where not merely the intellect but the whole person is implicated in the process, any serious prac-titioner will seek out, value, and be grateful for the counsel of an adept.

Of course, we must examine our teachers carefully before we com-mit to them, just as any teacher worth his or her salt will scrutinize prospective disciples with great care before taking on the huge re-sponsibility of teaching. It is also clear that as the *guru* tradition takes root in our modern world, it will undergo a certain degree of change. In particular, it is likely to lose some of its paternalistic fla-vor. But regardless of this change, the challenge for the disciple will always be to drop the ego baggage and cultivate genuine humility, discipline, and an eagerness to learn and go beyond the present level of understanding and attainment until mastery is achieved.

The mass media have profitably manipulated public opinion by muddling up the *guru* tradition with the emotionally charged phe-nomena of cult leadership and brainwashing. It will be a long time before a more truthful picture can emerge. But the age-old, well-tested Yoga tradition, which has great vitality, will easily survive pub-lic opinion. Furthermore, as the more flamboyant and questionable teachers drop out of sight as the students themselves become more realistic and mature, Yoga will very likely gain in strength over the years to come.

We can only hope that in the course of this natural evolution more and more Yoga practitioners will discover the authentic teachings, which are fulfilled by the great adepts. As students become more educated about genuine Yoga, they will also more readily recognize the genuine teachers.

Who are those teachers? They are the ones who are living proof of the validity and efficacy of the yogic teachings, who have mastered the ego and realized the Self and are demonstrating in their daily life the great virtues of wisdom and compassion, patience and generosity, and freedom from fear and anger. They are capable of deeply transforming their disciples, guiding them skillfully to the same sublime realization. They are an utterly benign power in the world.

There is no doubt that our world is in dire need of the nectar of wisdom flowing from those who have transcended the ego-personality and realized the Self and whose only concern is the enlightenment of others. The drone of our technological civilization has largely deafened us to their voices. But they continue to gift us with their wisdom and their spiritual presence. All we need to do to benefit from their incessant transmission of light is to become quiet and listen to our own hearts. This is where Yoga begins, unfolds, and fulfills itself.

Notes

Chapter 1: Introducing Yoga

1. This is the revised and enlarged edition of my earlier book *Yoga: The Technology of Ecstasy* (Los Angeles: Jeremy Tarcher, 1986).

Chapter 2: The Principal Branches of Yoga

1. Swami Vivekananda, *Jnana-Yoga*, rev. ed. (New York: Ramakrishna-Vivekananda Center, 1982), p. 12.
2. R. Powell, ed., *The Ultimate Medicine: As Prescribed by Sri Nisargadatta Maharaj* (San Diego, Calif.: Blue Dove Press, 1994), p. 39.
3. Ibid., p. 65.
4. Ramana Maharshi, *Forty Verses on Reality: Ulladu Narpadu*, transl. S. S. Cohen (London: Watkins, 1978), pp. 32–33.
5. See, for example, *Brihad-Aranyaka-Upanishad* IV.2.4.
6. I. P. Sachdev, *Yoga and Depth Psychology* (Delhi: Motilal Banarsidass, 1978), p. 129.
7. S. N. Dasgupta, *Hindu Mysticism* (Chicago: Open Court, 1927), p. 126.
8. The word *brahman* is derived from the verbal root *barh*, meaning "to increase, expand, strengthen." In its original Vedic sense of "prayer," *brahman* means that inner activity that swells with strength until one becomes one with the Absolute, also called *brahman* in later times.
9. M. Eliade, *Patanjali and Yoga* (New York: Schocken Books, 1975), p. 10.
10. B. K. S. Iyengar, *The Tree of Yoga* (Boston: Shambhala Publications, 1989), p. 106.

161

Chapter 3: The Teacher, the Disciple, and the Path

1. Cited in T. M. P. Mahadevan, *Ramana Maharshi: The Sage of Arunacala* (London: Mandala Books, 1977), p. 180.
2. See G. Feuerstein, *Holy Madness: The Shock Tactics and Radical Teachings of Crazy-Wise Adepts, Holy Fools, and Rascal Gurus* (New York: Paragon House, 1991).
3. D. Rudhyar, *Directives for New Life* (n.p.: Ecology Center Press, 1971), p. 44.
4. Ibid.
5. U. Arya, *Mantra and Meditation* (Honesdale, Pa.: Himalayan International Institute, 1981), p. 147.

Chapter 4: Happiness and the Moral Foundations of Yoga

1. The Sanskrit text does not distinguish between "oneself" and "Self"—in both cases the word *atman* is used. Therefore this sentence can also be rendered as "One should lift oneself by oneself." However, in the final analysis, it is the transcendental Self that allows one to break through the conditioning of the self, or ego-personality. At least this is the metaphysical position espoused in the *Bhagavad-Gita*.
2. T. Roszak, *Unfinished Animal: The Aquarian Frontier and the Evolution of Consciousness* (London: Faber & Faber, 1976), p. 213.
3. Ibid.
4. Sri Aurobindo, *A Practical Guide to Yoga* (Pondicherry, India: Sri Aurobindo Ashram, 1955), p. 209.
5. Swami Sivananda, *Practice of Yoga* (Sivanandanagar, India: Yoga Vedanta Forest Academy Press, 1970), p. 69.

Chapter 5: Purification and Postures for Relaxation, Meditation, and Health

1. The word *nirvana* means "extinction" and refers to the transcendence of the ego in the moment of enlightenment.
2. See A. Berger and J. Berger, *Reincarnation: Fact or Fable?* (London: Aquarian Press, 1991); J. Head and S. L. Cranston, eds. *Reincarnation: An East-West Anthology* (Wheaton, Ill.: Quest Books, 1985).
3. M. Eliade, *Yoga: Immortality and Freedom* (Princeton, N.J.: Princeton University Press, 1973), p. 54.

4. Sri Aurobindo, *The Synthesis of Yoga I/II* (Pondicherry, India: Sri Aurobindo Ashram, 1971), p. 29.
5. B. K. S. Iyengar, *Light on Yoga* (New York: Schocken Books, 1976), p. 98.
6. Sri Aurobindo, *Synthesis*, p. 30.
7. M. V. Bhole, "Viscero-Emotional Training and Re-Education through Yogasanas," *Yoga-Mimamsa* 19, nos. 2 and 3 (1977–1978), p. 47.
8. The word *khecari* is composed of *khe* ("in the ether/space"—*kha*) and *cari*, from *car* ("to move").

Chapter 6: Yogic Diet

1. R. Ballentine, *Diet and Nutrition: A Holistic Approach* (Honesdale, Pa.: Himalayan International Institute, 1978).
2. *Young India*, August 8, 1921, p. 261.
3. *Young India*, October 7, 1946, p. 347.
4. *Harijan*, February 2, 1949, pp. 430–431.
5. O. M. Aivanhov, *The Yoga of Nutrition* (Frejus, France: Prosveta, 1982), p. 38.
6. Ibid., pp. 14–15.
7. Ibid., p. 17.

Chapter 7: The Breath: Secret Bridge to Vitality and Bliss

1. However, many other Vedanta authorities, including the famous Badarayana (who composed the *Brahma-Sutra*), equate the *ananda-maya-kosha* with the transcendental Self.
2. Swami Vivekananda, *Complete Works of Vivekananda*, vol. 1, pp. 143–144, quoted in Swami Prabhavananda, *The Spiritual Heritage of India* (Hollywood, Calif.: Vedanta Press, 1979), p. 252.
3. Paramahansa Yogananda, *Autobiography of a Yogi* (Nevada City, Calif.: Crystal Clarity, repr. 1994), p. 236.
4. Swami Rama, *Lectures on Yoga: Practical Lessons on Yoga* (Honesdale, Pa.: Himalayan International Institute, 1979), p. 93.
5. S. Dasgupta, *Hindu Mysticism* (Chicago: Chicago University Press, 1927), p. 75.
6. See G. Krishna, *Kundalini: The Evolutionary Energy in Man* (London: Robinson & Watkins, 1971). This edition has an introduction by Frederic Spiegelberg and a psychological commentary by James Hillman.

7. T. Bernard, *Hatha Yoga: The Report of a Personal Experience* (London: Rider, 1971), p. 58.
8. Ibid., p. 95.

Chapter 8: Pathways of Concentration and Meditation

1. Swami Nikhilananda, *Hinduism: Its Meaning for the Liberation of the Spirit* (New York: Ramakrishna-Vivekananda Center, 1972), p. 138.
2. See J. Varenne, *Yoga and the Hindu Tradition* (Chicago: University of Chicago Press, 1976), p. 118.
3. See Swami Muktananda, *Play of Consciousness (Chitshakti Vilas)* (San Francisco: Harper & Row, 1978).
4. J. Blofeld, *The Tantric Mysticism of Tibet* (New York: E. P. Dutton, 1970), pp. 84–85.
5. U. Arya, *Superconscious Meditation* (Honesdale, Pa.: Himalayan International Institute, 1977), p. 80.

Chapter 9: Sacred Sounds of Power: Mantras

1. A. Govinda, *Foundations of Tibetan Mysticism* (London: Rider, 1969), pp. 27–28.
2. Swami Ramdas, *At the Feet of God* (Bombay: Bharatiya Vidya Bhavan, 1977), p. 35.
3. Ibid., p. 3.
4. Sir J. Woodroffe, *The Garland of Letters: Studies in the Mantra-Śastra* (Madras: Ganesh, repr. 1974), p. 228.

Chapter 10: The Serpent Power: Kundalini Shakti

1. G. Krishna, *Kundalini*, pp. 12–13.
2. Ibid., pp. 51–52.
3. G. Krishna, *The Real Nature of Mystical Experience* (New York: New Concepts Publishing, 1978), p. 28.
4. L. Sannella, *The Kundalini Experience: Psychosis or Transcendence?* (Lower Lake, Calif.: Integral Publishing, 1987), p. 154.
5. Swami Muktananda, *Secret of the Siddhas* (South Fallsburg, N.Y.: SYDA Foundation, 1980), p. 11.

6. R. E. Svoboda, *Kundalini: Aghora II* (Albuquerque, N.M.: Brotherhood of Life, 1993), pp. 66–67.
7. Western writers often take the syllables *ha* and *tha* to be the actual Sanskrit words for "sun" and "moon," which is wrong.
8. See M. Govindan, *Babaji and the 18 Siddha Kriya Yoga Tradition* (Montreal: Kriya Yoga Publications, 1991).

Chapter 11: Tantra-Yoga: The Transmutation of Sexual Energy

1. A. Watts, *Nature, Man, and Woman* (New York: Vintage Books, 1970), pp. 187–188.
2. B. Bhattacharya, *The World of Tantra* (New Delhi: Munshiram Manoharlal, 1988), p. 377.

Chapter 12: Self-Transcendence, Ecstasy, and Freedom

1. Sri Aurobindo and The Mother, *A Practical Guide to Integral Yoga* (Pondicherry, India: Sri Aurobindo Ashram, 1955), p. 146.
2. See Bubba Free John, *The Enlightenment of the Whole Body* (Middletown, Calif.: Dawn Horse Press, 1978).
3. G. Feuerstein, *Wholeness or Transcendence? Ancient Lessons for the Emerging Global Civilization* (Burdett, N.Y.: Larson Publications, 1992), p. 169.
4. J. C. Pearce, *The Bond of Power: Meditation and Wholeness* (London: Routledge & Kegan Paul, 1982), p. 155.
5. Ibid., p. 156.
6. A. Alston, *Yoga and the Supreme Bliss* (London: A. Alston, 1982), pp. 50–51.
7. Here the plural noun *yogas* stands for *yogins*.
8. G. Heard, *Training for the Life of the Spirit* (London: Cassell, 1944), pp. 57–58. This is a booklet.
9. P. Brunton, *The Notebooks of Paul Brunton*, vol. 13, *Relativity, Philosophy, and Mind* (Burdett, N.Y.: Larson Publications, 1988), p. 209.
10. Ibid., p. 189.

Chapter 13: Yoga in the Modern World

1. C. G. Jung, *Psychology and the East* (Princeton, N.J.: Princeton University Press, 1978), p. 85.
2. Ibid.
3. H. Jacobs, *Western Psychotherapy and Hindu Sadhana* (London: George Allen & Unwin, 1961), p. 153.

Recommended Publications

In addition to the publications referred to in the endnotes, the reader may also profit from consulting the following books and periodicals.

Books

Aivanhov, Omraam Mikhael. *The Yoga of Nutrition.* Frejus, France: Prosveta, 1982.

———. *Man's Subtle Bodies and Centres.* Frejus, France: Prosveta, 1986.

———. *The Powers of the Thought.* Frejus, France: Prosveta, 1988.

———. *"Know Thyself": Jnana Yoga.* Parts 1 and 2. Frejus, France: Prosveta, 1992–1993.

Arya, U. *Mantra and Meditation.* Honesdale, Pa.: Himalayan International Institute, 1981.

Aurobindo, Sri. *On Yoga.* Pondicherry, India: Sri Aurobindo Ashram, 1957.

———. *On Yoga II: Letters on Yoga.* Pondicherry, India: Sri Aurobindo Ashram, 1969.

———. *The Synthesis of Yoga.* Pondicherry, India: Sri Aurobindo Ashram, 1976.

Avalon, A. (John Woodroffe). *The Serpent Power.* New York: Dover Publications, 1974.

Ayyangar,T. R. S. *The Yoga Upaniṣads.* Adyar, India: Adyar Library, 1952.

Brunton, P. *The Hidden Teaching beyond Yoga.* New York: Samuel Weiser, 1972.

———. *A Search in Secret India.* New York: Samuel Weiser, 1977.

———. *The Notebooks of Paul Brunton.* 16 vols. Burdett, N.Y.: Larson Publications, 1984–1988.

Bubba Free John. *The Paradox of Instruction.* San Francisco: Dawn Horse Press, 1977.

166

————. *The Enlightenment of the Whole Body*. Middletown, Calif.: Dawn Horse Press, 1978.

Criswell, E. *How Yoga Works: An Introduction to Somatic Yoga*. Novato, Calif.: Freeperson Press, 1989.

Eliade, M. *Yoga: Immortality and Freedom*. Princeton, N.J.: Princeton University Press, 1973.

————. *Patanjali and Yoga*. New York: Schocken Books, 1975.

Evans-Wentz, W. *Tibetan Yoga and Secret Doctrines*. London: Oxford University Press, 1971.

Feuerstein, G. *Introduction to the Bhagavad-Gita: Its Philosophy and Cultural Setting*. Wheaton, Ill.: Quest Books, 1983.

————. *The Yoga-Sutra of Patanjali*. Rochester, Vt.: Inner Traditions, 1990.

————. *Sacred Paths*. Burdett, N.Y.: Larson Publications, 1991.

————. *Wholeness or Transcendence? Ancient Lessons for the Emerging Global Civilization*. Burdett, N.Y.: Larson Publications, 1992.

————. *The Shambhala Encyclopedia of Yoga*. Boston: Shambhala Publications, forthcoming. A revised and enlarged edition of *Encyclopedic Dictionary of Yoga*, first published in 1990.

————, and S. Bodian, eds. *Living Yoga: A Comprehensive Guide for Daily Living*. Los Angeles: J. P. Tarcher, 1993.

————, Subhash Kak, and David Frawley. *In Search of the Cradle of Civilization*. Wheaton, Ill.: Quest Books, 1995.

Frawley, D. *Tantric Yoga and the Wisdom Goddesses*. Salt Lake City, Utah: Passage Press, 1994.

Ghosh, S. *The Original Yoga*. Delhi: Munshiram Manoharlal, 1980. A translation of the *Shiva-Samhita*, *Gheranda-Samhita*, and *Yoga-Sutra*.

Govindan, M., ed. *Thirumandiram: A Yoga Classic by Siddhar Thirumoolar*. Translated by B. Natarajan. Montreal: Babaji's Kriya Yoga and Publications, 1993.

Iyengar, B. K. S. *Light on Yoga*. New York: Schocken Books, 1976.

————. *Light on Pranayama*. New York: Crossroad, 1981.

————. *The Tree of Yoga*. Boston: Shambhala Publications, 1989.

Krishna, G. *Kundalini: The Evolutionary Energy in Man*. London: Robinson & Watkins, 1971. With a psychological commentary by James Hillman.

————. *The Biological Basis of Religion and Genius*. London: Turnstone Press, 1973.

————. *The Riddle of Consciousness*. New York: Kundalini Research Foundation, 1976.

————. *Living with Kundalini: The Autobiography of Gopi Krishna*. Edited by Leslie

Shepard. Boston: Shambhala Publications, 1993. An expanded edition of *Kundalini* (1971), without the Hillman commentary.

Kriyananda, Swami. *The Path: Autobiography of a Western Yogi*. Nevada City, Calif.: Ananda Publications, 1977.

Mishra, R. S. *Fundamentals of Yoga: A Handbook of Theory, Practice, Application.* New York: Julian Press, 1959.

Muktananda, Swami. *Play of Consciousness (Chitshakti Vilas)*. San Francisco: Harper & Row, 1978.

Radhakrishnan, S., trans. *The Bhagavadgita*. London: Routledge & Kegan Paul, 1960.

———. *The Principal Upanisads*. London: Allen & Unwin/New York: Humanities Press, 1974.

Rieker, H. U. *The Yoga of Light*. Los Angeles: Dawn Horse Press, 1973. A translation of and commentary on the *Hatha-Yoga-Pradipika*.

Sannella, L. *The Kundalini Experience*. Lower Lake, Calif.: Integral Publishing, 1987.

Śivananda Radha, Swami. *Kundalini: Yoga for the West*. Spokane, Wash.: Timeless Books, 1978.

———. *Radha: Diary of a Woman's Search*. Spokane, Wash.: Timeless Books, 1981.

———. *Hatha Yoga: The Hidden Language*. Spokane, Wash.: Timeless Books, 1987.

———. *Mantras: Words of Power*. Spokane, Wash.: Timeless Books, 1994.

Subramuniyaswami, S. Satguru. *Dancing with Śiva: Hinduism's Contemporary Catechism*. Concord, Calif.: Himalayan Academy, 1993.

Varenne, J. *Yoga and the Hindu Tradition*. Chicago: University of Chicago Press, 1976.

Venkatesananda, Swami. *The Concise Yoga Vāsiṣṭha*. Albany, N.Y.: SUNY Press, 1984.

Vishnudevananda, Swami. *The Complete Illustrated Book of Yoga*. New York: Crown, 1988.

Vivekananda, Swami. *Jnana-Yoga*. Rev. ed. New York: Ramakrishna-Vivekananda Center, 1982.

———. *Karma-Yoga and Bhakti-Yoga*. New York: Ramakrishna-Vivekananda Center, 1982.

———. *Raja-Yoga*. New York: Ramakrishna-Vivekananda Center, 1982.

Wilber, K. *The Spectrum of Consciousness*. Wheaton, Ill.: Quest Books, 1977.

———. *The Atman Project*. Wheaton, Ill.: Quest Books, 1980.

Yogananda, Paramahansa. *Autobiography of a Yogi*. Nevada City, Calif.: Crystal Clarity, 1994.

Zvelebil, K. V. *The Poets of the Powers.* Lower Lake, Calif.: Integral Publishing, 1993. An introduction to the Yoga of the South Indian Siddhas.

Magazines

Hinduism Today. A monthly newspaper published by the Himalayan Academy. Editorial offices: 1819 Second Street, Concord, CA 94519. Subscription address: P.O. Box 157, Hanamaulu, HI 96715. Tel.: (800) 822-1008 or (808) 822-3152.

Inner Directions Journal. A quarterly magazine published by Inner Directions. P.O. Box 231486, Encinitas, CA 92023. Tel.: (619) 471-5116.

Intuition. A quarterly magazine published by Colleen Mauro. P.O. Box 460773, San Francisco, CA 94146. Tel.: (415) 949-4240.

The Quest. A quarterly magazine published by the Theosophical Society in America. Editorial offices: P.O. Box 270, Wheaton, IL 60189-0270. Subscription address: P.O. Box 3000, Denville, NJ 07834-3000. Tel.: (800) 669-9425.

Shambhala Sun. A bimonthly magazine founded by Chögyam Trungpa Rinpoche. P.O. Box 399, Halifax Central, Halifax, N.S. B3J 2P8, Canada. Tel.: (902) 422-8404.

Tantra: The Magazine. A quarterly magazine published by Alan Verdegraal. P.O. Box 10268, Albuquerque, NM 87184. Tel.: (505) 898-8246.

Yoga International. A bimonthly magazine published by the Himalayan International Institute. Rural Route 1, Box 407, Honesdale, PA 18431. Tel.: (717) 253-6241.

Yoga Journal. A bimonthly magazine published by the California Yoga Teachers Association. Editorial offices: 2054 University Avenue, Berkeley, CA 94704. Subscription address: P.O. Box 469018, Escondido, CA 92046-9018. Tel.: (510) 841-9200.

Useful Resources

Books

Integral Publishing
P.O. Box 1030
Lower Lake, CA 95457
(for books by Georg Feuerstein)

Prosveta U.S.A.
P.O. Box 49614
Los Angeles, CA 90049
(for books by Omraam Mikhael Aivanhov)

South Asia Books
P.O. Box 502
Columbia, MO 65205
Tel.: (314) 474-0116
Fax: (314) 474-8124
(for hard-to-get books published in India;
catalogue available upon request)

Yoga Journal's Book and Tape Resource
2054 University Avenue
Berkeley, CA 94704-1082
Tel.: (800) 359-9642

Hatha-Yoga and Meditation Supplies

Dharmacrafts
405 Waltham Street, #234
Lexington, MA 02173
Tel.: (617) 862-9211
Fax: (617) 862-8824
(statues, cushions, bells, incense,
  books, videos, etc.; catalogue
  available upon request)

Harmony in Design
2050 S. Dayton
Denver, CO 80231
(inversion tables and backbend
  benches; $3.00 for color brochure)

Shasta Abbey Buddhist Supplies
P.O. Box 199
Mount Shasta, CA 96067
Tel.: (916) 926-6682
(statues, props, posters, incense,
  rosaries, books, and tapes; catalogue
  available for $2.00)

Yoga Studio
P.O. Box 415
Georgetown, CA 95634
Tel.: (800) 366-4541
(green sticky mats)

Organizations

International Association of Yoga
  Therapists
209 Hillside Avenue
Mill Valley, CA 94941
(Publishes newsletter and journal and
  operates a book club)

Yoga Research Center
P. O. Box 1386
Lower Lake, CA 95457
Tel.: (707) 928-9898
Fax: (707) 928-4738
Email: *yogaresrch@aol.com*
(Directed by Georg Feuerstein, the
  Center offers a variety of programs
  and publishes the bimonthly
  newsletter *Yoga World* and
  translations of Yoga texts.)

American Sanskrit Institute
73 Four Corners Road
Warwick, NY 10990
Tel.: (914) 986-8652
Fax: (914) 987-7097
(Directed by Vyaas Houston, the
  Institute offers courses and
  immersion training in Sanskrit, as
  well as cassettes and CDs.)

International Yoga Studies
Southwest Campus
13833 South 31st Street
Phoenix, AZ 85048
Tel.: (602) 759-1972
(Directed by Sandra Summerfield
  Kozak; conducts high-level Yoga
  teacher training and certification
  programs.)

Index